Reducing the Risks for
Substance Abuse
A Lifespan Approach

D0782981

PREVENTION IN PRACTICE LIBRARY

SERIES EDITOR

Thomas P. Gullotta
Child and Family Agency, New London, Connecticut

ADVISORY BOARD

George W. Albee, University of Vermont
Evvie Becker, University of Connecticut
Martin Bloom, University of Connecticut
Emory Cowen, University of Rochester
Roger Weissberg, University of Illinois
Joseph Zins, University of Cincinnati

HIGH-RISK SEXUAL BEHAVIOR:
Interventions with Vulnerable Populations
Evvie Becker, Elizabeth Rankin, and Annette U. Rickel

REDUCING THE RISKS FOR SUBSTANCE ABUSE:
A Lifespan Approach
Raymond P. Daugherty and Carl Leukefeld

SUCCESSFUL AGING: Strategies for Healthy Living
Waldo C. Klein and Martin Bloom

TYPE A BEHAVIOR: ITS DIAGNOSIS AND TREATMENT
Meyer Friedman

Reducing the Risks for Substance Abuse

A Lifespan Approach

Raymond P. Daugherty

Prevention Research Institute
Lexington, Kentucky

Carl Leukefeld

Multidisciplinary Research Center on Drug and Alcohol Abuse
Lexington, Kentucky

Plenum Press • New York and London

Library of Congress Cataloging-in-Publication Data

Daugherty, Ray.
    Reducing the risks for substance abuse : a lifespan approach /
Raymond P. Daugherty, Carl Leukefeld.
        p.   cm. -- (Prevention in practice library)
    Includes bibliographical references and index.
    ISBN 0-306-45898-5 (hc.). -- ISBN 0-306-45899-3 (pbk.)
    1. Alcoholism--United States--Prevention. 2. Drug abuse--United
States--Prevention. 3. Behavior modification--United States.
4. Life cycle, Human--United States.   I. Leukefeld, Carl G.
II. Title. III. Series.
HV5279.D38 1998
362.29'17'0973--dc21   98-29801
                                                            CIP

ISBN 0-306-45898-5 (Hardbound)
ISBN 0-306-45899-3 (Paperback)

© 1998 Plenum Press, New York
A Division of Plenum Publishing Corporation
233 Spring Street, New York, N.Y. 10013

http://www.plenum.com

10 9 8 7 6 5 4 3 2 1

Printed in the United States of America

Every idea and every word that we have contributed to this book have been formed by the years of partnership, and friendship, with Terry O'Bryan, co-founder of Prevention Research Institute. Only illness kept her from co-authoring this work and nothing short of having her name on the cover could adequately express the impact she has had on its development, and on Lifestyle Risk Reduction in general. Even in her illness, she continues to be an inspiration to many—but most especially to us.

—R. P. D. and C. L.

Preface

Join Us on a Prevention Mapping Expedition

The real difficulty, the difficulty that has baffled the sages of all times is rather this: how can we make our [prevention] so potent in the emotional life of people, that its influence should withstand the pressures of the elemental psychic forces in the individual?

—Albert Einstein

The challenge of prevention is to change human behavior in a way that will keep problems from occurring. But how do we make prevention programs powerful enough not only to change behaviors, but also to maintain that change over time? In our opinion, there is no single answer to this question, and answers, as well as related questions, will continue to evolve. But the prevention journey has begun and progress has been made. In many ways, though, it is a journey in which more theoretical routes exist than those that are tried and true. Few have been to the desired destination (achieving sustained behavior change), and those who have only succeeded in finding paths that work for a part of the population. Clearly, maps are being drawn and revised as we go.

Viewed from this perspective, prevention is an exploration—and a mapping expedition—into a largely unknown territory.

As with any such expedition, we expect to find that a number of initially promising paths will not take us where we intended and must be abandoned. Other paths will get us close to the goal but will need revision. Still, if we learn from the journey, and map it clearly so others can follow productive paths and avoid pitfalls, there is no complete or absolute failure. Learning is progress, even if the outcome is different from what we hoped.

This book proposes new prevention paths, revises old ones, and suggests abandoning several current popular paths that do not appear to be moving us in the right direction. This may be troubling for some readers. If so, we encourage patience at the difficult times, and an explorer's mindset, coupled with an appreciation for new possibilities. Every explorer faces similar barriers: examining the tides of accepted beliefs, navigating currents of anxiety, and bracing for the winds of resistance. Sometimes those barriers come from outside, sometimes from within. In either case, we believe that we must be persistent, flexible, and willing to entertain new thoughts. The task of obtaining and maintaining behavior change has, after all, "baffled the sages of all times." If we are going to make progress, it is our opinion that we must be willing to question our most basic assumptions. This could be painful for some and liberating for others.

Perhaps there is no assumption more fundamental to alcohol and drug abuse prevention than the belief that the primary focus is, and should be, youth. This would at least seem to be the focus in the United States since about 1980. Current alcohol and drug abuse prevention programs are so inherently youth-focused that most discussions of prevention assume the target audience is youth. "Prevention" and "prevention for youth" are, for the most part, treated synonymously. In fact, it is our observation that most alcohol and drug prevention theories are based on youth data and only address prevention for young people. As a reflection of this, most books, curricula, and other alcohol and drug abuse prevention materials are designed with the assumption that elementary, middle school, or high school age students are the target audience. Most materials developed for adults (such as a parent or teacher) are intended to help them accomplish prevention among youth. Furthermore, there is such a lack of prevention theory and materials for any other part of the lifespan that prevention efforts directed at other age groups are generally designed for youth and applied to adults, often with mixed results. More importantly, in youth-focused prevention, the assumptions and decisions that affect prevention actions are made based on what is true for childhood and adolescence, generally with little or no consideration for the rest of the lifespan. The motto seems to be: "If it is good for kids, it is good for prevention." While there is an inherent appeal to this way of thinking, it only seems valid for issues specific to childhood and not those carried forward into adulthood. For lifetime issues, we generally measure success of prevention programs by how well children have been prepared for the rest of their lives. In our opinion, there is reason to believe that the youth focus has led to prevention that is short-lived for youth, sometimes counterproductive as young people mature into adulthood, and generally irrelevant to adults.

Since there seems to be a natural tendency to think in opposites, we quickly suggest that the alternative to youth-focused prevention is not adult-focused prevention, but lifespan-focused prevention. In lifespan-focused prevention, every decision is made within the context of the whole lifespan. Consideration is given not only to how the prevention activity will affect the target audience at their current age, but also how it will affect them at future ages. Thus, prevention programs aimed at any age should make sense and have relevancy at all points in the lifespan so prevention is not counterproductive in any age group. In no way does a lifespan approach mean abandoning youth, though it may change what we say and do with young people. Prevention with youth should actually become stronger in a life-span focused approach since young people will understand more clearly how the behavior expected of them fits in with behaviors expected of adults, and they will continue to find the prevention message relevant and useful at each age level. But many steps must be taken before we can fully explain what lifespan-focused prevention means. We will begin by asking basic questions about the nature of the alcohol and drug problem to determine whether the prevention map should, in fact, be limited to the years of youth or be broadened to include the lifespan.

We invite you to join us in this mapping expedition.

Acknowledgments

We sincerely thank Jill Crouch for the days of work she invested in editing and document preparation. We also thank Phillip High for illustration and Diane Bobys for document preparation. We are also deeply indebted to a number of people who provided excellent review and comment on a very tight schedule. This includes Possie Raiford in Georgia; Allan Barger, Doris Morrow, and Mark Nason in Kentucky; Tom Frostman in Colorado; Rick Kritzer and Allison Sharer in Ohio; and Deb Synhorst in Iowa. Thank you.

Contents

Chapter 1. Mapping Prevention: For Childhood or the
            Lifespan?   1

Chapter 2. Rethinking Prevention from a Lifetime Perspective 23

Chapter 3. A Foundation for Lifespan-Focused Prevention .. 49

Chapter 4. Learning from Youth-Focused Prevention Models 71

Chapter 5. Behavior: The Ultimate Risk and Protective
            Factor   95

Chapter 6. Maximizing Behavior Change 115

Chapter 7. Special Issues in Lifestyle Risk Reduction 143

Chapter 8. Concluding Remarks 159

References 163

Index 171

About the Authors 177

1

Mapping Prevention
For Childhood or the Lifespan?

"Which way should I go?" said Alice. "That depends on
where you want to end up," replied the cat.
—Lewis Carroll, *Alice in Wonderland*

Maps provide paths and paths go to destinations. In a mapping
expedition, we do not have the luxury of a known path. The need
to know where we want to go, though, is at least as great when we
are drawing the map as when others are following it. Only in
knowing our ultimate destination can we assess the accuracy of the
path and make midcourse corrections. For prevention, this requires
a clear understanding of our target audience and what we want to
accomplish.

In the past couple of decades, we have asked hundreds of groups
the same question, "Who is the target audience for prevention?" The
most common reply is, "children." Both the general public and
prevention professionals seem to share that view. Current prevention
theory is grounded in research on young people and centered on
childhood and adolescence. Starting with the elementary ages, there
appears to be an inverse relationship between the availability of
prevention programs and the age of the audience. Federal agencies
now include a youth audience as part of the definition of prevention
(Office of Substance Abuse Prevention, 1991). Many decision mak-
ers establish prevention definitions, goals, and strategies based only

1

on how they impact youth. "Prevention" and "prevention with youth" have, for all practical purposes, become synonymous. If prevention is a mapping expedition, the journey seems to stop somewhere around age 21. We refer to this current reality as youth-focused prevention.

Advocates of youth-focused prevention generally rely on one or more of four assumptions: (1) Alcohol and drugs are primarily a youth problem; (2) age of first use defines prevention as a youth issue; (3) use at a young age causes problems later; and (4) youth-focused prevention has been successful. But should we be mapping prevention for childhood or for the lifespan? An examination of the four assumptions can help provide the answer.

ARE ALCOHOL AND DRUGS PRIMARILY A YOUTH PROBLEM?

Many people believe that drug and alcohol use is heaviest among young teens. In reality, for all abused substances other than inhalants, ages 12–17 have a lower rate of use than the 18–25, 26–34, or 35+ age groups (U.S. Department of Health and Human Services, 1996). For alcohol, use-related problems are higher among young adults and adults, peaking in the 18–25 age group and again in the 35+ age group. The highest rate of abuse and dependence of illegal drugs is in the 18–29 age group (Anthony & Helzer, 1991). As shown, both use and problems occur throughout the lifespan, with the highest rates in the young adult or adult years. Therefore prevention strategies are needed throughout the lifespan. Prevention activities for young people should have an enduring impact into adulthood.

DOES AGE OF FIRST USE DEFINE PREVENTION AS A YOUTH ISSUE?

Another rationale for youth-focused prevention is that use begins at a young age. Statistically, if people do not use drugs prior to a certain age, they are very unlikely to ever use. Some people also believe that it is too late for prevention once use begins. There is no doubt that initiation of alcohol and drug use occurs at a young age, though this is often overstated. For example, it is not unusual to read that people take their first drink at age 12–13. The *Monitoring the Future* study does indicate 12.9 as the average age of first use. However, this only applies for 12–17-year-olds *who drink* (Johnston, O'Malley, & Bachman, 1996). This data does not include those who begin drinking at an older age. Naturally, the younger the age of the group examined, the younger the age of first use will be as a function of simple math. For example, the age of first use among fourth graders who drink would be much younger than that of high school seniors who drink. According to the National Household Survey, which takes users of *all* ages into account, the average age for first use of alcohol is age 17. For cigarettes, it is age 15; inhalants, age 16; marijuana, age 18; heroin, age 20; cocaine, age 21; and tranquilizers, age 23 (U.S. Department of Health and Human Services, 1996). By considering all ages, the household survey gives a better indication of the entire population. However, it does obscure the fact that the age of first use has fallen over time. For example, the age of first use among those aged 18–25 is lower than for those age 35 or higher.

There is little doubt that if people do not smoke, drink, or use drugs by a certain age, they are much less likely to ever use. Some believe this is because young people are more easily influenced by peers. It could also be simply an issue of getting past the socially determined age of initiating the behavior, or perhaps past the age of rebellion. After a certain age, almost everyone who would consider using alcohol or drugs has done so. Many of those who are still abstainers by that age are adamantly against use and would not use at any age. Others may be curious and might yet sample drugs under the "right" circumstances, but they are unlikely to ever do more than sample. These same points are no doubt true for many social behaviors. People who have never danced, gone to a party, or played baseball by a certain age are also not likely to do so at any age. It is likely that a significant number of people would only initiate use of certain substances during adolescence. According to the Centers for Disease Control and Prevention, for example, 91 percent of all adult smokers began smoking before age 20. Since the majority of adults do not smoke, it seems reasonable to assume that most of those who make it to age 20 without smoking are not likely ever to smoke. If we properly support abstinence during these years, initiation of use is unlikely. This fact provides logical support for increasing the rate of abstinence among young people. However, this does not rule out the need for prevention at other ages, especially for alcohol.

DOES EARLY USE CAUSE LATER PROBLEMS?

In 1989, the Office (now Center) for Substance Abuse Prevention published, as its first monograph, a report of the Committee on the Future of Alcohol and Other Drug Use Prevention of the Institute for Behavior and Health, Inc. (Dupont, 1989). The report cites data indicating that people who use at the youngest ages are most likely to experience alcohol and drug problems later. The committee was firm in using this as a rationale for youth-focused prevention. The inherent logic is appealing and simple. Stop use early and you stop problems later.

A number of studies (Kandel, 1982) indicate that those who are drinking the most and experiencing problems with alcohol or drugs as young adults are likely to have begun their use at a younger age than others. Also, those who have their first Driving Under the Influence (DUI) arrest at a younger age are more likely to have a second DUI than those who have their first DUI at older ages. Robins and Przybeck (1985) found that people who begin drug use before the age of 15 are almost twice as likely to experience use-related problems as those who initiate use after the age of 19.

A 1998 article provided even clearer support for a link between age of beginning use and later development of problems. Grant and Dawson (1998) conducted a study using data from the National Longitudinal Alcohol Epidemiological Survey. This survey involved face-to-face, retrospective interviews with 42,862 people, age 18 and older. Of the 27,000 people who drank, 20 percent had qualified at some time in their life for a DSM-III diagnosis of alcohol dependence. Another 7.4 percent qualified for a diagnosis of alcohol abuse. However, the percentage varied greatly based on the age at which the person began drinking. Of those who began drinking at age 13, 47.3 percent qualified for a diagnosis of alcohol dependence and 11.5 percent had qualified for a diagnosis of alcohol abuse at some point in their lives.[1] These figures dropped to 16.6 percent and 7.8 percent for those who began drinking at age 18. They dropped further to 9.5 percent and 4.9 percent for those who began drinking at age 22. However, contrary to the trend of lower problems with later onset of use, there was an increase in alcohol dependence to about 14 percent for those who began drinking at age 23 or 24.

Research has quite clearly established that people who begin using alcohol or drugs at a young age are more likely to experience problems related to use. Thus, proponents of youth-focused prevention logically assume that early use is a risk factor and that stopping use by young people would reduce later problems. However, Grant and Dawson (1998) commented on the danger of that assumption:

> Although these results suggest that preventive efforts should be targeted toward the delay of alcohol use onset until after ages 18 or 19 when the associated risk of alcohol abuse and dependence has dramatically dropped, such a recommendation should be considered cautiously. . . . The weakness of such a prevention strategy is the lack of a complete understanding as to why the onset of alcohol use is related to the development of alcohol abuse and alcohol dependence. (pp. 108–109)

They went on to say that more research is needed to

> ascertain if it is the delay in alcohol use or, *more likely* [emphasis ours], other associated factors that account for the inverse relationship between age at first drink and the risk of lifetime alcohol use disorders. Within this paradigm, another central research question is to determine

---

[1] This does not mean that this percent currently qualified for an alcohol dependence diagnosis. It means that during a one year period at some time in their life, they showed enough symptoms to qualify for this diagnosis. They may or may not have still showed those symptoms at the time the research was conducted. Also, this does not imply that a diagnosis was ever made. Many people qualify for a DSM-III alcohol abuse or dependence diagnosis at some time in their lives, but do not continue having problems.

the status of early onset use as either a critical and potentially modifiable risk factor in the development of alcohol use disorders, or alternatively, as a marker or early indicator of the . . . development of alcohol use disorders. (p. 109)

In other words, it is likely that people in our culture who begin drinking at age 15 or younger differ in important ways from people who begin drinking at age 21. By age 15, only 13.5 percent of Americans who will ever drink have begun drinking. By age 21, however, 85.3 percent of those who will ever drink have begun drinking. In other words, anyone drinking before or after these ages is equally "out of sync" with the norms. They may be out of sync because of social, emotional, or biological differences, difficulties, or problems. These differences could account for both the early and the late users being out of sync with other users and for their increased rate of problems. As early as 1974, Cahalan and Room (1974) noted that people who drink, but come from a group for whom drinking is not normative, are much more likely to exhibit problems with alcohol. They suggested that people who engage in one socially "deviant" behavior (different from the norm) may differ from the norm in other ways that make them prone to problems.

Both the early use and the increased risk for problems may result, then, from some third factor or set of factors. If this is the case, age of first use would be *predictive* of later problems, but would not *cause* the problems. This has real implications for prevention. If early use is the cause of later problems—a risk factor—then raising the age of use would lower the rate of problems at a future age. On the other hand, if early use is a sign of impending problems—a risk indicator (or marker), not a risk factor—then delaying the age of first use is not likely to reduce later problems. Instead, early use may best serve as a "flag" to identify people who need intensive prevention to address the "other" issues that lead both to early use and later problems. The danger is that if prevention programs approach a risk marker as a risk factor, we may miss the real issue, thus reducing effectiveness. Research seems to support the position that age of use is a marker of risk, not a risk factor. For example:

- A number of the studies showing that early use predicts later problems find that those who experience problems began using only a few months before their peers. If age itself is the key issue, then it is hard to imagine that beginning use at age 9.5 versus 10.2, for example (Samson, Maxwell, & Doyle, 1989), is going to be meaningful. Is age itself the issue, or is there something different about people who are the "first users," regardless of age?

- The average age of first use changes from time to time. When it changes, the age at which a person is an "early user" also shifts. It is relative. Early users from one decade may be older than early users from another decade. Yet, regardless of the specific age, the principle does not seem to change. Early users still experience more problems than later users. If age of first use itself increases the risk for later problems, this should not occur. For example, if drinking or using drugs before age 15 increased risk because of age itself, then as the average age of first use drops below age 15, the rate of problems should increase proportionately. That does not seem to occur. Instead, as age of first use drops, the age at which "early use" predicts later problems also drops. This suggests that "use before one's peers" is the real issue, regardless of what that age happens to be. If that is the case, then it is likely that a third factor may be responsible for both the early use and the later problems.

- If age itself is a risk factor, then those who use at age 15 in one culture should experience similar risk to those who drink at age 15 in another culture. Also, cultures that routinely expose young people to alcohol should have very high rates of problems. This does not seem to occur. Instead, it has been clear for many years that some of those cultures seem to have lower rates of problems than our own (Plaut, 1967).

- There is also evidence that in cultures where drinking by youth is normative, early use still predicts later problems, though the age differs greatly. For example, a New Zealand study (Fergusson, Lynskey, & Horwood, 1994) found that those who began drinking prior to age six experience more problems than those who began drinking after age 12. There is a huge difference between age 6 in the New Zealand research and age 15 as was indicated in Robins and Przybeck (1985). Again, the issue does not appear to be age *per se*. The most relevant question appears to be, "What causes a young person to begin using prior to peers?"

- Robins and Przybeck (1985) found that among the younger people in their study, age of first use occurred before age 15 but was *less* predictive of later problems than among the older people in their study. These younger people grew up in a time when drug use was more nearly normative. As use becomes more nearly normative, early use becomes less predictive of later problems. This also suggests that there is nothing magical about age 15, or any other specific age. Drinking alcohol before age 15 (or any other age) may only be a significant predictor if a culture prescribes that drinking is not to occur at that age, and if most 15-year-olds do not drink. Once again, the data suggest that age itself is not the issue. Instead, people who "break the rules first" differ from the norm in some important ways, even when compared to people who break the rules later. These people are more problem prone. The correlation between early use and later problems has little to do with age. Instead, early use is a good way to identify people who are prone to breaking rules and getting in trouble. However, as breaking the rules becomes normative, those who break the rules no longer differ from the norm. The behavior loses clinical significance.

- There is also evidence (Anthony & Helzer, 1991) that *early initiation of use of illegal drugs* best predicts *problems at an early age*. Those who experience problems after age 29 are not as likely to show an early onset of use. A personal communication to Raymond Daugherty in January 1998 from Grant and Dawson revealed a similar finding for alcohol. Other research also shows that those who experience alcohol problems at an older age often had a short drinking history, beginning heavy use in the middle or older adult years (Sobell, Cunningham, Sobell, & Toneatto, 1993). It seems likely, then, that there are fundamental differences between people who experience problems at a young age and those who experience problems only at an older age.

• Some data also indicate that *older* initiation of use is more predictive of risk for alcoholism. Gomberg (1993) cites evidence that women who develop alcoholism average an older age of first use of alcohol than those who do not develop alcoholism. This trend has held up over several decades. In the 1960s, the same trend was observed among males who developed alcoholism (Plaut, 1967). Grant and Dawson's (1998) data indicated that both early and late use were associated with increased rates of alcohol dependence. Together, these findings seem to argue that age itself is not the real issue.

A closer look at the Robins and Przybeck data (1985) seems to also support the conclusion that some third factor increases the likelihood of both early use and later problems. Their data did indicate that those who began drug use before age 15 were more likely to develop drug problems later. However, it also showed that these young people had a high level of panic attacks and depressive symptoms *before they began using drugs. This group was also more likely to have both alcoholic and antisocial relatives.* Both of these factors show up time and again in the research.

Kubicka, Kozeny, and Zdenek (1990) found that age of first use was predictive of later problems only for people with a family history of alcoholism. Research also indicates that children of alcoholics who develop alcoholism do so about 10 years earlier than those without a parent who has alcoholism. They also begin drinking (Chassin et al., 1991) and experiencing drinking-related problems (Goodwin, 1984) at a younger age. Children of alcoholics are also more likely to have a low P3 brain wave and preadolescent boys with a low P3 are more likely to drink prior to age 16 (Berman et al., 1993). In addition, individuals with antisocial personality disorder (ASP) tend to begin drinking and using drugs at a younger age. Those with ASP who develop alcoholism do so about 10 years younger than those who have alcoholism and do not also have this disorder (Hesselbrock et al., 1984). This group not only uses more drugs and alcohol, but is also prone to more trouble. Hesselbrock and colleagues provide data indicating that when the two conditions overlap, the ASP contributes most to early onset of use, and family history of alcoholism contributes most to negative consequences of drinking. Penick et al. (1987) found that early onset alcoholics were more likely to have a family history of alcoholism, ASP, or other coexisting psychiatric problems. Cloninger's "Type 2" alcoholics appear to have a family history of alcoholism and antisocial personality disorder. An early age of onset and multiple legal and social problems characterize Type 2 alcoholism (Cloninger, Bohman, & Sigvardsson, 1981).

There is a great deal of evidence, then, that those who drink or use drugs prior to their peers are different from their peers in some important ways. They even differ from other users who begin at an older age. Those who develop alcoholism early are also different in some important ways from those who develop alcoholism later. They are more likely to have family histories of alcoholism or antisocial tendencies. They are also more likely to have emotional problems, conduct disorder, antisocial personality disorder, or to be highly rebellious. These factors influence the person to "break the rules" and begin using before peers. This could create the illusion that use at a younger age leads to a greater likelihood of problems. In fact, it seems more likely that these other factors contribute to both the younger age of use and to the increased rate of problems.

Other psychological and social factors also seem to influence the decision to use alcohol or drugs at an early age. For example, young people who score higher on indicators of rebellion are also prone to drink earlier, use illicit drugs earlier, and violate laws and social norms while using (Kandel, 1982). Seventh graders who drink and engage in other deviant behaviors or have poor grades are more likely to be binge drinking in the eighth grade (Ellickson & Hays, 1991). High sensation-seeking has been linked to early use and to increased problems. Several studies have shown that youth who drink at a young age were exposed to more peers and adults who drink. Both factors, especially exposure to peers who use marijuana, are predictive of heavier alcohol use (Ellickson & Hays, 1991).

Together, these findings seem to support the conclusion that age of first use may be more an *indicator* of impending problems than a *cause* of impending problems. Early users are not typical of the total population of users.

A final possibility is that all of the above factors are true and each explains part of what occurs. We believe that is likely. It seems reasonable that age could be directly linked to increased problems. However, these differences would most likely be found by comparing onset of use at markedly different ages. For example, a person who begins using marijuana or alcohol at age 13 may be more likely to experience psychological dependence or behavioral problems than a person whose first use is at age 20. This alone would argue that one prevention goal should be to delay the onset of use. However, outcomes that are associated with initiating use only a few months, or even a year or two, before one's peers seem less likely to be age related. It seems more reasonable that these are situations in which some other factor is contributing to the person being a first user, a heavy user, and a problem user. This may include personality variables such as rebelliousness or antisocial personality; social variables such as peer group and socioeconomic status; and, possibly, biological variables such as family history of alcoholism. Delaying the age of first use is an important goal, but will not solve the problem by itself, nor does it support a prevention approach that is predominantly youth focused. Prevention programs for younger ages are not the only prevention needed.[2]

---

[2] A related question is whether those who make high-risk choices and have problems at a young age are likely to maintain the behavior into adulthood. The apparent answer is both yes and no. Wechsler and Isaac's (1992) research with college students indicates that a significant percentage of high-risk college drinkers were likely to have been high-risk drinkers in high school as well. Of course, there was also a significant percentage of college high-risk drinkers who were not high-risk drinkers in high school.

Separate studies conducted by Cahalan and Room (1974) with multiple national samples, by Vaillant (1995) with a 50-year longitudinal study, and by Fillmore, Bacon, and Hyman (1979) following up Straus' Drinking in College Sample, all reported that a significant percentage of high-risk college-age drinkers are likely to be making high-risk drinking choices and experiencing problems even two and three decades later. But high-risk use does not necessarily carry forward from one age to another. In each of these studies, an equal or larger percentage of young people who experienced serious alcohol problems at college age changed their drinking behavior and "grew out of it." Thus, high-risk behavior begets high-risk behavior, but prevention of some sort (with or without a formal prevention program) also happens at a variety of ages, including the adult years.

HAS YOUTH-FOCUSED PREVENTION BEEN SUCCESSFUL?

Use Decreased among Youth in the 1980s

To answer this question, we must look at the results of prevention efforts during the 1980s and 1990s. These were the watershed years of youth-focused prevention. By the end of the 1980s, it appeared that youth-focused prevention was a resounding success. A significant prevention effort, launched with a combination of government and private funding, was followed by a marked drop in alcohol and drug use by adolescents. Marijuana and alcohol use by high school seniors were both about 20 percent lower in 1993 than in 1979. The percentage who sometimes drinks 5 or more drinks in a row decreased from 41 percent in 1979 to about 28 percent in 1992 (Johnston et al., 1996). Overall, the percentage of Americans who reported use of any illicit substance decreased from almost 25 percent in 1979 to about 12 percent in 1994. This translates to a decrease from 24 million to 12 million drug users. The number of new cocaine users dropped from about a million and a half in 1980 to half a million in 1992. Between 1975 and the early 1990s, the number of new heroin users also dropped by 25 percent. Alcohol-related traffic fatalities in 1993 were almost half what they were a decade earlier.

Use Increased among Youth in the 1990s

However, as has been consistent with drug and alcohol use patterns throughout U.S. history, the pendulum of use seems to be swinging once again. There has been an increase in drug use among teens that generally began in 1992 for 8th graders, and in 1993 for 10th and 12th graders. For inhalants, the increase began to show up in 1987 for high school seniors. The largest increase is for marijuana use, although teen use of hallucinogens and cocaine has also increased. Heroin use is up among both teens and adults. There was also a slight increase starting in 1994 and 1995 for 12th graders who reported having five or more drinks in a row. In short, there are reasons to conclude that prevention programs were working among teens in the 1980s but are not working as well in the 1990s.

High-Risk Drinking Increased among Adults

There are also reasons to conclude that prevention programs have worked less well for adults. The percentage of Americans age 21 and older who abstain from alcohol has increased since 1979. However, *high-risk drinking* has also increased among adults, primarily for those age 21–34. Consistent with this change, the percentage of adult males who reported diagnostic symptoms of alcohol dependence also increased (Clark & Hilton, 1991; Hasin, Grant, Harford, Hilton, & Endicott, 1990).

Alcohol-Related Death Rate Increased

Changes in the types of alcohol-related deaths show a dual pattern. There have been significant decreases in DUI deaths, with the greatest decrease in younger drivers. It is not clear whether this decrease is due to a change in drinking behavior or driving behavior. Designated drivers allow a decrease in crashes without a decrease in drinking. Driving deaths aside, the overall rate of alcohol-induced deaths *increased* by more than 8 percent between 1979 and 1992. This again implies an increase in high-risk drinking among adults.

College Age: Abstinence, High-Risk Drinking, and Problems All Increased

The high school students in the above data grew up with no-use prevention. The adults did not. Youth-focused prevention did not attempt to reach adults, but it did promise that drug-free youth would grow into drug-free adults. The sharp decline in drinking among high school students between 1979 and 1993 provides an excellent opportunity to examine the validity of this promise. If it is true, there should have been a decline in alcohol use as these high school students entered college. A two-part study done by Wechsler and Isaac (1992) sheds light on this. Their research measured the drink-

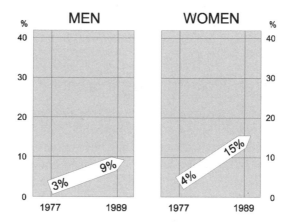

Figure 1.1.   Abstaining in college 1977–1989.

ing of first-year college students on a number of different campuses, first in 1977 and again in 1989.[3] The 1977 students went through junior high and high school during years of "responsible use" prevention and accelerating use. The 1989 students grew up during the years of "no-use prevention" and declining use. Wechsler and Isaac's findings were both remarkable and troubling.

Between 1977 and 1989, the percentage of first-year college students who abstained from alcohol tripled among men and quadrupled among women (see Figure 1.1). By itself, the data on absti-

[3]Some comments about vocabulary may be helpful before looking at data. First, in examining data on drinking, it is important to make distinctions between drinking (consuming any amount of alcohol) and high-risk drinking (consuming amounts of alcohol that significantly increase one's risk for problems). The reasons for this will become very clear as we look at data. Also, drawing upon data from multiple studies is challenging because various researchers define terms differently or use different terms to describe the same behavior. We have done our best to simplify this for the reader. We will use the terms "low-risk choices," "high-risk choices," and "problem outcomes" (which are defined in Chapter 4) throughout this book. When we use the term "high-risk drinking" when describing various research findings, the definition used in the particular study may not coincide exactly with the definition we will use in Chapter 4, but will always be high-risk. For example, researchers frequently measure "five or more drinks in a row," which is also called "binge drinking," or "heavy episodic drinking." That is above the amount we will define as being high-risk, thus while "five or more drinks" should be seen as high-risk, it does not imply that a lower amount is necessarily low-risk. Whenever we refer to data on "drinking," we are including both high-risk and low-risk drinking.

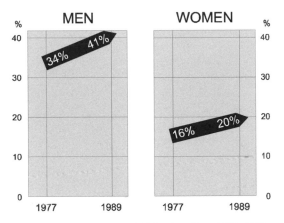

Figure 1.2. High-risk drinking in college 1977–1989.

nence supports the promise of youth-focused prevention: Higher rates of abstinence in high school carried forward into college.

However, between 1977 and 1989, there was also a 20 percent increase in high-risk drinking among men and a 25 percent increase for women (see Figure 1.2). The percentage who got drunk 1–3 times in the previous month went up by two-thirds for men and two-and-a-half times for women (see Figure 1.3). The percentage who drank specifically for the purpose of getting drunk doubled

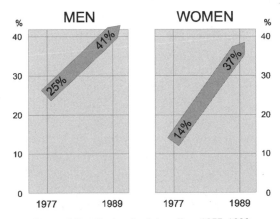

Figure 1.3. Getting drunk in college 1977–1989.

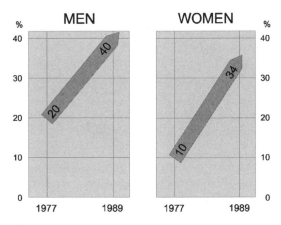

Figure 1.4.   Drinking to get drunk in college 1977–1989.

among men and increased three-and-a-half times among women
(see Figure 1.4).

Predictably, while abstinence and high-risk drinking increased, low-risk drinking decreased. Wechsler and Isaac (1992)
observed that light drinking was "disappearing" from the college
campus. They further commented that the college freshmen in 1989
had gone through high school during the height of the "Just Say No"
prevention implementation. What can this tell us about the long-
term impact of youth-focused prevention?

Wechsler and Isaac (1992) did not collect data from these college
students as high school seniors. However, nationally the high school
senior class of 1988 had a higher rate of abstinence and a lower rate
of high-risk drinking compared to the senior class of 1976 (Johnston
et al., 1996). Wechsler and Isaac's data indicate that, a year later as
college freshmen, the rate of abstinence was still higher for the 1980s
group. This is consistent with one promise of youth-focused prevention, but contrary to another promise: Their rates of high-risk drinking
and problems were also higher. It would be tempting to laud the
continued increase in abstinence and downplay the increase in high-
risk use. Overall, though, college students had greater risk of experiencing alcohol-related problems in 1989 than in 1977.

This research does not stand alone. Schuckit, Klein, Twitchell,
and Springer (1994) compared drinking of college students in 1980

and 1992 and found that, while the rate of abstinence had increased, the rate of problems had also increased. For example, the percentage experiencing memory blackouts increased from 22 percent to 40 percent; missed school or work from 15 percent to 25 percent; "shakes" from 9 percent to 17 percent; and binges from 8 percent to 16 percent. Once again, while the years of exposure to the no-use message increased abstinence, it did not lower the rates of high-risk drinking and problems among college students. Instead, these increased.

Monitoring the Future data is not fully consistent with the above. These data show a decrease in the percentage of college students reporting five or more drinks in a row. Perhaps the difference in these findings lies in the different definitions, measures, and sampling procedures used.[4] However, other studies have had findings similar to Wechsler and Schuckit. Also, research on cocaine indicates that this trend is not limited to alcohol.

Cocaine: Fewer Users—More Use and More Problems

According to the National Household Survey, the number of new cocaine users dropped from almost one-and-one-half million in 1980, to just over a half million in 1993 (U.S. Department of Health and Human Services, 1996). From 1979 to 1994, the percentage of the population that used cocaine dropped from about 4 percent to

[4] Schuckit was measuring problems and Wechsler and Isaac were measuring a higher level of high-risk drinking than was *Monitoring the Future*. (Wechsler and Isaac used the same measure as *Monitoring the Future* in a later analysis, but they did not include any time comparisons.) The measure of five or more drinks per day that is used by *Monitoring the Future* is of limited value with college students because so many students drink much larger quantities. In our own work, we measure up to "13 or more drinks" on an occasion. It is possible, for example, that the discrepancy in the findings could be explained by a reduction in those drinking five or six drinks as their peak amount, but an increase in the peak by those drinking more. If this occurred, it would account for the decrease in five or more in *Monitoring the Future* as well as the increase in heavier drinking and in problems found in the other studies. It is also possible that sampling procedures could explain the differences. The *Monitoring the Future* sample is a subset of their high school sample which may or may not be representative of college students in general.

just over 1 percent. From the perspective of no-use prevention, this is a great success. Yet during this same period, the total amount of cocaine used in the United States increased from 150 metric tons to almost 300 metric tons! According to a study done by the RAND Corporation (Everingham & Rydell, 1994), the reason seemed to be a large increase in the number of heavy users. In 1979, about two-thirds of the cocaine used in America was consumed by casual users and one-third was consumed by "hard-core" users. By 1994, these figures had more than reversed so that one-fourth of the cocaine users consumed two-thirds of the nation's cocaine supply. As a result of this shift from light to heavy use, health consequences of cocaine use have gone up significantly. Nationwide, cocaine-related emergency room admissions went up from about 1000 in 1979 to about 140,000 in 1994 (McCaig et al., 1996).

Are These Changes Related to Youth-Focused Prevention?

The era of youth-focused, no-use prevention has been associated with an increase in abstinence at all ages and a decrease in high-risk use for high school age students. It has also been associated with an increase in high-risk drinking and alcohol-related problems for those above high school age. Determining whether these changes result from youth-focused prevention is difficult at best.

Patterns of alcohol and drug use are in constant fluctuation. Thus, it is possible that the increases in abstinence were a societal trend unrelated to prevention efforts. Decreases in drug use had already begun before initiation of the 1980s "War on Drugs." In addition, a significant increase in abstinence among adults preceded the increases in abstinence among the young.

Population trends may also explain some of the changes in use. Drug use decreased at the same time that the teen population decreased. Use is now increasing at the same time that the teen population is increasing. A larger population may provide greater anonymity for illegal behaviors. It may also expose each young person to a larger number of drug users, even if the percentage does not change. Thus, a bulge in population could create the illusion of increased use, which then leads to an actual increase in use. A reduction in population might reverse the process. Though this theory is consistent with research showing that misperceptions of peer use affect actual use, it is still speculative.

However, several facts support the possibility that the reduction in teen use is, at least to some extent, a result of youth-focused prevention. While the reductions in adolescent drug use began before the launch of the most recent War on Drugs, these reductions greatly accelerated after the campaign was in place. This suggests that the prevention efforts may have increased the magnitude of the change even if they did not initiate it. Also, reductions in high-risk alcohol use by teens did not begin until after the prevention campaign had been in place for several years. This also suggests that sustained effort made a difference. In addition, youth-focused prevention had been in place and growing for a few years prior to the War on Drugs. One could argue that as youth-focused prevention came into widespread use, rates of teen use began to drop. As youth-focused prevention grew into the War on Drugs, larger reductions in use among teens began to occur.

A type of "backdoor" support also comes from the fact that prevention of the 1980s targeted youth and largely ignored adults. The reductions that occurred in high-risk use of alcohol among teens were not mirrored in the adult population. In fact, high-risk drinking and related problems actually increased among adults. A decade of decreases occurred in the young audience that was targeted, while high-risk use and problems actually increased in the adult group that was not targeted.

Additional support comes from *Monitoring the Future* data. Teens' perception that marijuana use is dangerous increased for a couple of years before marijuana use declined in the 1980s. Bachman, Johnston, and O'Malley (1988) argued persuasively that these changes were the result of more realistic, risk-focused marijuana education. If they are correct, it would mean that the no-use prevention succeeded in reducing marijuana use. This raises a second interesting possibility. A decreased perception that marijuana is hazardous preceded the 1990s increase in marijuana use. If changes in prevention could explain the positive changes during the 1980s, could other prevention changes explain the later increases in use?

This seems possible. Late in the 1980s, theories driving youth-focused prevention became more generic. In response, federal and state prevention agencies began promoting prevention that was less substance specific. Congress supported this by allowing Drug-Free Schools money to be spent on violence, teen pregnancy, and AIDS prevention. Schools and prevention agencies began moving away from drug-specific education. This relates to Bachman et al.'s (1988) suggestion that realistic marijuana education led to changes in attitude and reductions in use. If they are correct, then the move away from drug-specific prevention may have allowed antiuse attitudes to decay and use to increase.[5]

Taken together, the above data provide evidence that youth-focused prevention may indeed have succeeded in increasing abstinence, and even in reducing high-risk use among high school students. However, its impact was short-lived. The increases in teen use could be related to prevention becoming more generic. Other possible reasons for these increases will be explored in the next chapter. If we only look at young people, there is reason to believe that youth-focused prevention did work and that returning to intensely implemented, drug-specific implementation of youth-focused prevention would work again. Broadening our vision beyond high school students, however, underscores the major problems with this approach. The era of youth-focused prevention has been accompanied by a decrease in use by youth, but, an increase in high-risk use and problems among young adults and adults. Most importantly, youth-focused prevention appears to fail to keep one of its most important promises. As young people move from high school to college, the rates of high-risk drinking and problems go up, even though the rate of abstinence also increases.

---

[5] During the 1996 presidential campaign, the increase in teen drug use became a major issue, with each political party blaming the other. In fact, many within the prevention field who were watching the data predicted that an increase in use was coming based on the decreases in perceived risk that were occurring. These decreases, and even the predictions, happened prior to the 1992 change of presidential power. Clearly, the forces that were driving this go beyond which party was in the White House since they spanned two administrations. It is important to realize that perception of risk is such a powerful predictor of behavior, even among teens, that it afforded behavior changes to be accurately predicted.

CONCLUSION

The supporting assumptions of youth-focused prevention seem to be flawed. Drug use is not a problem unique to youth; it is a problem that covers the lifespan. Clearly, those who do not begin use in their teen years are not as likely to ever use. But does this in any way argue for prevention to be exclusively youth-focused? We think not. While there is reason to begin prevention early, there is no reason to stop it early. The broader areas of health promotion and disease prevention have many examples of successful prevention activities for adults. Further, data show that alcohol and drug use and related problems are greatest among young adults and adults. This means prevention is needed at all ages.

Advocates of youth-focused prevention claim that early use increases the risk for experiencing problems later in life. However, the data they use to support this claim really show that those who use prior to their peers are more likely to experience problems, regardless of age. These early users differ from late users in some important ways. It seems likely that both the early use and the later problems share the same root cause. Early use, then, is a predictor of problems, but is probably not the cause of the problems.

Proponents of youth-focused prevention have also maintained that increasing abstinence among teens will reduce problems in adulthood. Instead, data indicate that no-use prevention does increase the rate of abstaining in college, but is also associated with an increase in high-risk drinking and problems. Similarly, the number of cocaine users has decreased dramatically, but the amount of cocaine used has increased. As a society we must decide whether we want—indeed, whether we can afford—to support a prevention approach that does not prepare young people for a lifetime. Even more so, can we afford to continue to support a prevention approach that appears to contribute to increasing high-risk use at the very ages that already had the highest rate of high-risk use?

There is an alternative.

2

Rethinking Prevention from a Lifetime Perspective

> We can't change unless we completely rethink what it is
> we are doing, unless we have a wholly new vision of what
> we are doing.
>
> —John Naisbitt, *Megatrends*

Changing our thinking from a youth focus to a lifetime focus requires more than simply broadening the target audience. When we limit our thinking to a specific age group, we make different assumptions and arrive at different conclusions than when we expand our vision to include the lifespan. Each conclusion and each assumption help form prevention goals, messages, activities, programs, and policies. The age-limited assumptions that currently guide prevention have led us down paths that have not been as productive as any of us would have liked. This chapter examines a few of the most important areas in which this seems to have occurred. We believe the conclusions that logically follow a lifespan focus will ultimately be more effective for youth, adults, and society. To assist in considering the issues, we will pose three questions: (1) What are we trying to prevent? (2) Is a no-use approach the most effective prevention strategy? (3) How do we design prevention to grow with youth?

WHAT ARE WE TRYING TO PREVENT?

To know the purpose of prevention, we must answer the question, "What are we trying to prevent?" Other fields define the purpose of prevention as keeping *problems* from developing. If problems did not occur, there would be no need for prevention. For example, the purpose of heart disease prevention is to keep related illnesses, deaths, and costs from occurring. Strategies to prevent those problems include increasing exercise, decreasing smoking, and decreasing dietary fat intake. It is not likely that heart disease professionals would turn this around to say that they are really trying to prevent sedentary lifestyles and high-fat diets.

However, this reversal is exactly what has happened in alcohol and drug abuse prevention since the introduction of youth-focused prevention. Quotations from several U.S. Government publications illustrate this shift. In 1983, *Prevention Plus* (National Institute of Alcohol Abuse and Alcoholism, 1983) described the purpose as "preventing alcohol and drug *problems*." A separate monograph implied a similar goal in its title, *Preventing Adolescent Drug Abuse* (Glynn, Leukefeld, & Ludford, 1983). In 1989, the foreword of *Prevention Plus II* (Office of Substance Abuse Prevention, 1989) described the purpose of prevention as, "the *use* of any illegal drugs, the illegal *use* of alcohol, and the *use* of legal drugs in ways they were not intended." However, the "definitions" section still defined the objective of primary prevention as being "to avoid problems." It went on to say that the terms "alcohol abuse prevention" and "drug abuse prevention" should not be used "except when referring to adults." By 1991, *Prevention Plus III* (Office of Substance Abuse Prevention, 1991) described prevention only in terms of preventing use by teens. In less than a decade, what we are trying to prevent shifted from "problems" and "abuse" to "use," and the population served became limited to youth.

Many people now accept prevention of use as the intrinsically true, unquestionable definition of prevention, rather than as just one particular philosophy. Sometimes people support this by saying that use *is* the problem. However, that is like saying high-fat diets are the problem instead of heart disease. On one level, it has truth. On a larger level, it misses the point. Before the late 1800s, most drugs were legal and widely viewed as sources of good, rather than evil. Since drugs were not recognized as harmful, there were no drug prevention efforts. Only recognition of a problem stimulates interest in prevention. Once the problems generate enough concern, people use various prevention strategies to eliminate or reduce whatever is leading to the problem. As we will see, defining the purpose of prevention as "preventing use" can sometimes work against reducing problems.

Our field redefined the purpose of prevention after rejecting the ill-conceived "responsible use" approach (National Institute on Alcohol Abuse and Alcoholism, 1977). That approach had dominated prevention in the 1960s and 1970s, and may have contributed to increased use. When one approach is rejected, it is often replaced by its opposite. In this case, "no-use" prevention provided the greatest possible distance from "responsible use" prevention. Advocates of this change reasoned that any focus on reducing problems might support a continued focus on responsible use. Redefining the purpose of prevention as preventing use removed any possibility that prevention strategies might imply acceptance of use. Applying the no-use message to alcohol made it necessary to either seek a return to Prohibition or exclude adults from prevention. Focusing only on youth avoided challenges from adults who did not want a return to prohibition or a challenge of their own use of alcohol. Thus, defining prevention of use as the purpose simultaneously defined youth as the only practical target audience for prevention. This age restriction is the first problem created by the redefinition of the purpose of prevention.

Another problem is that use, once it begins, is no longer a prevention issue. An article on drug use among athletes (Carr, Kennedy, & Dimick, 1996) illustrates this point. It suggested that prevention "is designed to dissuade athletes from using drugs altogether, before the experimental stage." Intervention, it suggested, is "necessary following confirmation that an athlete has tested positive for the first time for using an illegal substance." The article goes on to say that treatment was for those who "have a serious drug problem requir(ing) specialized, intensive help." How do we prevent problems in the rather large group who are beyond experimental use, but who have not been caught or exhibited some other problem? This is an important oversight. We do not mean to imply that this exclusion is purposeful, but neither is it uncommon or limited to prevention among athletes. It is simply the logical oversight of an approach that does not include all the necessary variables.

When a problem involves high-risk behaviors, prevention focuses on people who engage in those behaviors. Heart disease prevention focuses on people who have high-fat diets and sedentary lifestyles. Traffic safety efforts focus on people who speed, drive carelessly, or do not wear seat belts. Alcohol and drug prevention is an exception. If reduction of high-risk behaviors is a major prevention issue in all other fields, why is it not so in the alcohol and drug field?

Defining our purpose as preventing use instead of problems has obscured the clarity of our purpose. Only by virtually ignoring prevention for adults has this position been maintained as long as it has without major challenge. How are we to be successful in prevention programs for adults if the only goal is to prevent use? Are only adult abstainers in the prevention audience? Do adults who have one glass of wine with dinner need intervention? For that matter, we can ask the same questions regarding those under age 21. The only lifetime prevention position that is consistent with the "no-use" approach would be a return to Prohibition. Indeed, youth-focused prevention has been functioning in an environment of age-specific prohibition. When we expand our thinking to include the lifespan, it becomes clear that these assumptions no longer work. That does not mean that we should accept use by teens or return to the days of "responsible" drinking prevention as some have advocated (Milgram, 1996). It does mean that the definition of prevention needs to work for all substances and all ages. We might have different goals and different strategies for different ages, but the definition should work for all. Once we broaden our prevention thinking to recognize that prevention requires not only increasing abstinence, but also reducing high-risk use, surprising discoveries await us.

IS THE "NO-USE" APPROACH THE MOST EFFECTIVE PREVENTION STRATEGY?

There are two views on the source of alcohol and drug problems. The first view maintains that problems come from the general pool of users and any reduction in the percentage of users will lead to a reduction in problems. In this view, abstinence is always the best strategy to prevent problems. The assumption is that if young people abstain until age 21, they are likely to abstain forever. This no-use approach is central to youth-focused prevention. The first monograph of the Center for Substance Abuse Prevention clearly articulated this position (Dupont, 1989). The committee writing the monograph even felt that delaying the onset of use implied acceptance of use. Thus, they firmly held to nonuse as the only prevention goal. People also refer to this approach as "zero tolerance" or "abstinence only." Most of us are familiar with its "Just Say No" and "Drug-Free" slogans.

This view treats risk as an on-and-off switch. Use creates risk and nonuse turns off risk. This position seems logical and is emotionally satisfying. It is obvious that a person who never uses drugs or alcohol will not experience use-related problems. It follows that, if we could be 100 percent successful in eliminating use, all problems would disappear. In the real world, though, it is rare to eliminate behaviors that many people enjoy. It is not clear whether modest increases in nonuse will adequately reduce problems.

The second view treats risk as more of a dimmer switch. This view maintains that most problems do not come from the general pool of users. Instead, most problems come from the subgroup of heavy users, and the heavier the use, the greater the risk. The most effective way to reduce problems is to either increase abstinence or reduce high-risk use among these high-risk users. Reducing the general pool of users will lead to a reduction in problems only if we also reduce the subgroup of high-risk users. This view also assumes that some people in the general pool of users are more likely to become high-risk users. Others are very unlikely to become high-risk users. Thus, reductions in the general pool of users will reduce future rates of problems only if there has been a change in the behavior of those who are likely to become heavy users.

This second view guides the practice of most types of prevention. However, alcohol and drug abuse prevention has steadfastly held to the first view focusing on "high-risk youth" instead of "high-risk use." We believe that the data presented below gives strong support for the second view. These data lead to three conclusions about use and problems in the United States. First, people who make high-risk choices consume most of the alcohol and drugs.

Second, people who make high-risk choices experience most of the use-related problems. Third, the greatest potential for prevention is in reducing the highest-risk use.

The Heaviest Users Consume Most of the Alcohol and Drugs

High-risk drinkers consume most of the alcohol sold in the United States. While the lightest 10 percent of drinkers consume an average of two drinks each per *year*, the heaviest 2.5 percent of drinkers consume an average of 12 drinks each per *day* (Greenfield, Giesbrecht, & Kavanagh, 1996)! In fact, the lightest drinking two-thirds of all drinkers consume only 10 percent of the alcohol while the heaviest drinking one-third consumes 90 percent! (see Fig. 2.1). For cocaine, the data is similar. One-fourth of the cocaine users consumes two-thirds of all the cocaine used in the United States (see Fig. 2.2). Clearly, use of alcohol and drugs is not evenly distributed among users. Risk for problems is also not evenly distributed.

The Heaviest Users Experience Most of the Problems

In a very real sense, alcohol-related problems are not problems of drinking but of *high-risk* drinking. For example, the National

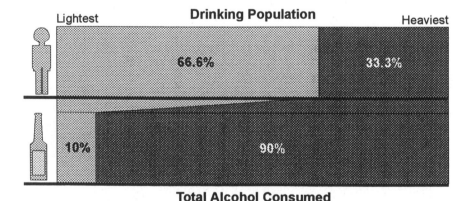

Figure 2.1.   The heaviest drinking third drinks 90 percent of the alcohol.

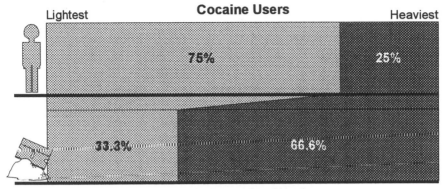

Figure 2.2. One-fourth of the cocaine users consumes two-thirds of the cocaine.

Household Survey asks questions about 18 different alcohol-related problems or problem indicators. These problems range from drinking in the morning to losing a job. Of those who reported never getting drunk, only 2 percent reported experiencing three or more problems. Of those who got drunk twice a month or less, 26 percent experienced three or more of the problems. Of those who reported getting drunk more than twice a month, 60 percent reported three or more of the eighteen problems. In the final analysis, virtually all alcohol-related problems occur as a result of high-risk drinking. Thus, levels of *high-risk* drinking are a more important prevention issue than levels of drinking.

Analyzing peaks that occur in drinking, high-risk drinking, and problems further illustrates this point. The percentage who drinks peaks in the 26–34 age group. If problems come primarily from the general pool of drinkers, then problems should peak in this age group. Instead, the peak age for alcohol-related problems is 18–25, which is also the peak age for high-risk drinking.

Prevention educators frequently state that "alcohol causes" any number of problems such as liver damage, driving fatalities, or job problems. In every case, though, there is a level of drinking below which these problems are rare and above which they become likely. Risk for problems is not an issue of drinking versus not drinking, it is an issue of quantity and frequency of drinking. This is even true for progression of use between substances.

Clearly there is a general progression of substance use. People do tend to use legal substances such as alcohol or tobacco before using illegal drugs. They also tend to use more accepted illegal drugs, such as marijuana, before using less socially acceptable illegal drugs such as cocaine. This has led to the "gateway drugs" concept which holds that use of one substance leads to use of another. For example, use of alcohol may lead to use of marijuana. Use of marijuana, in turn, leads to use of cocaine, and so forth.

Those who do not use alcohol are much less likely to use marijuana. However, a closer examination of the National Household Survey data (U.S. Department of Health and Human Services, 1996) shows that the relationship between alcohol and marijuana use is not a simple on-and-off switch. Of the 18–25-year-olds who drink alcohol, but never "binge" (drink five or more in one day), about 5 percent also use marijuana. The percentage more than triples among those who sometimes binge, and increases linearly with the frequency of binge drinking. Over half of those who binge ten or more times per month also use marijuana. The same trend is true for 12–17 year olds who drink. The younger group, though, passes the 50 percent mark at six episodes of binge drinking per month.

The same holds true for frequency of illegal drug use. Across the lifespan, only 0–3 percent of those who have used marijuana one to three times have also used cocaine, compared to 59–73 percent of those who have used marijuana more than 100 times (Clayton, 1984). Once again, it is not just use, but heavy use, that predicts progression to other drugs. This in no way implies that some use of marijuana may be low risk. It simply illustrates that quantity and frequency of use is a stronger predictor of other drug use.

No matter how we look at the data, we always come back to the same conclusions. Heavy users consume most of the alcohol and drugs and experience most of the problems. Risk is more like a dimmer switch than an on-and-off switch. What does this imply for prevention?

The Greatest Potential for Prevention

Where is the greatest potential to prevent problems? Does it lie in moving all of the lightest 10 percent of drinkers (who drink two drinks per year) to abstinence, or in persuading only a fraction of the heaviest one-third of drinkers (who drink 90 percent of all the alcohol) to reduce their drinking to within a low-risk range? The greatest potential to prevent problems lies in the reduction of high-risk use. In designing the most effective prevention campaigns for heart disease, such as the Stanford University Three Communities Study (Maccoby, Farquhar, Wood, & Alexander, 1977), people with the greatest risk get the highest priority. This should also be done in efforts to prevent alcohol and drug problems.

By definition, youth-focused prevention has eliminated this group from the prevention audience. We would not want to make the opposite error by implying that all of the heaviest-using population is in the prevention audience. Take, for example, the 33 percent of drinkers who consume 90 percent of the alcohol. For years, alcohol and drug educators have said that 10 percent of the drinking population has alcoholism. Some data indicate that the percentage is actually lower (Regier et al., 1990). However, if we accept this commonly used figure, then we can assume people with alcoholism comprise about 10 percentage points of this 33 percent. Prevention programs can still impact the remaining 23 percent who do not yet have alcoholism—if designed to meet the realities and the needs of the population.

To make this more concrete, imagine 10 drinkers drinking 100 cans of beer. If these 100 cans are consumed proportionately to how alcohol is consumed in the United States:

- Three of the people would share 90 cans of beer.
    - Of those three people, one person has alcoholism and needs a recovery program.
    - The other two people are high-risk drinkers who do not have alcoholism, but need prevention.
    - These two high-risk drinkers will experience numerous drinking-related problems.
- Seven people would share 10 cans of beer.
    - One of these seven people will only take a tiny sip.

Prevention programs may find it relatively easy to increase abstinence among the seven drinkers who shared 10 cans of beer. It may be especially easy to persuade the "tiny sip" person to abstain. (The "tiny sip" person represents the 10 percent of drinkers who average two drinks per year.) However, this will prevent virtually no problems unless there is a simultaneous decrease among the two high-risk drinkers who do not yet have alcoholism.

People who drink high-risk quantities, but do not have alcoholism, account for more problems than everyone else in the prevention audience combined. This group is not likely to respond to "Just Say No." They have been saying "yes" in a big way. We need different strategies to reach them, and we must use different measures of success. Returning to abstinence would be one measure of success, but not the only one.

In the last chapter we presented data for both alcohol and cocaine, suggesting that the abstinence-only prevention message was successful with the lightest users, but rejected by heavier users. It seems reasonable to assume that some of these "hard-core users" are dependent. We do a great injustice to our future, though, if we simply write this off as an intervention or treatment issue. *We need to ask how the number of high-risk users could rise so dramatically while the total number of users dropped so dramatically.* One possibility is that zero-tolerance prevention does nothing to reduce high-risk use among those who have the greatest interest in using. It only succeeds in supporting abstinence among those who have little interest in using. The only prevention goal has been to increase abstinence. No real effort has been made to persuade high-risk users of the need to reduce their use if they are unwilling to abstain. Of equal importance, no-use prevention does nothing to prevent *progression* to heavy use among those light users who reject the abstinence message. Youth-focused prevention only addresses abstinence. In this environment, use decreased and high-risk use increased. Since most problems come from the pool of heaviest high-risk users—not the total pool of users—problems also increased.

As noted, efforts to reduce high-risk use, and even efforts to delay the onset of use, have been rejected for fear they convey the message that use is acceptable (Dupont, 1989). While these fears seemed reasonable at the time, failure to reduce high-risk use has led to serious increases in heavy use and problems. In fact, there is evidence that failure to address high-risk use not only leads to more high-risk use in the long run, it may do so in the short run as well. For example, Ellickson and Bell reported in 1990 the results of a curriculum implemented with 7th graders that emphasized clear nonuse norms and social resistance skills. While there was some reduction in new smokers among program participants, there was actually an increase in smoking among those who smoked before being exposed to the curriculum. Again, we see the same pattern that occurred with general cocaine use and college students' alcohol use. The repeated pattern shows increases in abstinence accompanied by increases in high-risk use.[1]

[1] There is even reason to believe the national purchase age of 21 may have a dual impact based on age. There is a great deal of evidence indicating that the increase in purchase age decreased drinking and traffic fatalities among high school seniors and younger, at least for several years (Wagenaar & Streff, 1989). However, there is question about whether the law ever made a positive impact on those of college age. Hughes and Dodder (1992) conducted a longitudinal study of college drinking that surveyed student use of alcohol prior to passage of the national purchase age law, just after passage, and each semester for the following four years. They found that there was an increase in drinking just before the law was implemented, a decrease immediately after, and then a return to previous levels of drinking. They concluded that the law did not impact college drinking. Hughes and Dodder further noted that studies that followed the implementation of the law and did not have longitudinal data that predated implementation of the law were likely to erroneously conclude that the change in the law had reduced use. O'Hare (1990) reported that drinking and problems among college students under age 21 were at least as high as among those over 21, and noted that the law had only seemed to change the location of drinking for those under 21. A 1994 report of college drinking behavior (Allen, Sprenkel, & Vitale, 1994) documented that drinking—but not illicit drug use—was higher among college students who were under age 21. The researchers felt their findings were consistent with a rebellious backlash to the passage of the national 21 purchase age law, and cited other studies that they felt demonstrated the same (Allen et al., 1994). O'Malley and Wagenaar (1991) used the *Monitoring the Future* data to assess the effect of the 21 purchase age and also found a reduction in alcohol consumption at age 21. In addition, however, they found a "slightly" lower level of alcohol consumption among those age 21–25 who were raised in states that had a drinking age of 21. This later finding has been interpreted to mean that increasing the drinking age would lower drinking in the 21–25 age group (Center for Substance Abuse Prevention, 1997). However, it should be noted that O'Malley and Wagenaar were not measuring the impact of the change in the law. Their analysis was of a time period that preceded the change in the law, using states that had adopted the higher purchase age well before the national mandate to do so. The differences they measured could be due to the effect of a 21 purchase age or it could well be that differences in drinking attitudes and behaviors in those states led to both the lower level of drinking and the early adoption of a 21 purchase age. There are large variations in drinking patterns from state to state.

Other evidence also points to problems with the zero-tolerance approach as young people age. Researchers (Brown, D'Emidio-Caston, & Pollard, 1997) evaluating California's Drug, Alcohol, and Tobacco Education program (DATE) reported that, "as students matured, they increasingly responded to DATE programs with an apparently negative or indifferent affect, which increased from 10 percent (elementary school) to 33 percent (middle school) to over 90 percent at the high school level." The researchers also noted that, "Despite 25 years of cumulative evidence—found here in student's voices, and elsewhere in variable student substance-use rates, meta-analysis, and controlled studies all suggesting that students understand and reject the current no-use messages communicated in DATE (and similar) programs—many persist in delivering such programs" (pp. 79–80). They continued, "Let us be clear: we do not advocate programs promoting substance use. It is nonetheless becoming evident that our failures are not those of program implementation, but rather of program conceptualization and practice, and that the no-substance-use message contributes to drug education program failure."

It appears that youth-focused prevention has missed the mark on these issues. Logic argues that the purpose of prevention for the alcohol and drug field should be consistent with all other areas of prevention—to prevent problems. It is clear from the above data that large successes at increasing abstinence are not necessarily enough to prevent problems. Something else is needed.

Three Strategies Are Needed

We believe that prevention must pursue three strategies simultaneously: (1) increasing abstinence; (2) delaying the onset of use; and (3) reducing high-risk use. For certain audiences, increasing abstinence will be the most important prevention strategy. For others, reducing high-risk use will be the most important. To fail to reduce high-risk use is to fail at the prevention of problems, even if rates of abstinence have increased. Rates of abstinence must increase simultaneously with a decrease in high-risk use.

Some people are hesitant to accept reducing high-risk use as a prevention goal for young people. They do not want to give the message that use is acceptable (Dupont, 1989). This can be an emotional issue for those who interpret reduction of high-risk use to mean acceptance of use. Actively working to decrease high-risk use does not imply acceptance of use any more than working to decrease a high crime rate implies acceptance of crime. However, if we refuse to accept reduction of high-risk use as a goal, by default, we are accepting high-risk use. Obviously, we would prefer that no one use illegal drugs or high-risk quantities of alcohol at any time. However, our wishes do not dictate other people's choices.

Consider the following question, "Given that everyone is not going to abstain, is it better if those who refuse to abstain use large quantities of alcohol and drugs frequently or lesser quantities infrequently?" Those who choose the latter alternative have a position consistent with a prevention strategy to reduce high-risk use. However, it may take a while for the feelings to catch up with the position. It is important to realize that working to reduce high-risk use does not imply approval of use. It simply emphasizes the reality that if, as a society, we want to prevent alcohol and drug problems, we must actively work to reduce high-risk use *at the same time* that we are pursuing abstinence. We can accomplish this in a way that does not conflict with efforts to increase abstinence and does not confuse young people.

We agree with the DATE researchers that the problem is one of how prevention has been conceptualized. However, it is not the pursuit of abstinence that contributes to program failure, but the pursuit of abstinence without simultaneously pursuing reductions in high-risk use. The conceptual failure is in the unwillingness to address the lifespan with its complex needs and realities. There has also been a failure to conceptualize prevention theory, definitions, and strategies in ways relevant to the lifespan and to substances that are legal for adults. If by high school, 90 percent view prevention programs negatively, then prevention is losing its chance to be effective at the very ages when high-risk choices become likely. The prevention path has gone to an unintended destination. We need prevention that will grow with young people.

HOW DO WE DESIGN PREVENTION TO GROW WITH YOUTH?

Problems *do* occur and prevention *should* happen throughout the lifespan. The challenge is to design prevention so that it will "grow" with youth, remaining relevant as they grow into adulthood. Prevention strategies, concepts, and messages should be relevant to all points in the lifespan. At a minimum, prevention that "grows" with young people will prepare them for their futures, and not make them embarrassed about past prevention messages, behaviors, or attitudes. There are at least two difficult areas that we must address to accomplish this goal.

Making Sense of the Dichotomy of Legal Substances

Since prevention messages have been developed and delivered only with youth in mind, the messages have not made sense of the dichotomy of legal drugs. The basic message for youth has been, "Drugs are bad, just say no." This is an appropriate message for illegal drugs. People can relate to it for their whole lives. However, when we add a second message, "Alcohol is a drug," both children and adults become confused and prevention becomes less effective over time.

Consider a child in a family where there are no alcohol-related problems. The parents are part of the 70 percent of drinkers who drink only 10 percent of the alcohol. How is that child going to make sense of the message, "Alcohol is a drug, drugs are bad, do not use drugs?" Some children respond to this by saying, "Drugs are bad, alcohol is a drug, so my parents are bad, or are doing a bad thing." Parents have told us stories of their children crying, fearing that a parent is a "drug user." Some children plead with the parent to stop, pour out a parent's drink, or become upset at dinner when a parent has a single glass of wine. Remember, we are referring to low-risk drinking, not families where there is alcoholism or high-risk use. How will this same child react a few years later? If the child looks back with embarrassment, then drinking becomes an easy way to say, "I am no longer a silly little child." Prevention activities that are successful in elementary school, but cause embarrassment in high school, will be short-lived. These activities may ultimately provoke the behavior they tried to prevent.

Another immediate response from the young child may be, "Drugs are bad, alcohol is a drug, but my parents would not do anything really bad, so maybe drugs are not so bad after all." This unexpected response is not too far from the frequently heard argument, "You have your beer, why can't I have my pot?" Have youth-focused prevention messages inadvertently contributed to this argument? Could messages such as the ones we have just examined partially explain why youth-focused prevention has a 90 percent negative rating among high school students? Could it help explain why prevention appears to stop working by college age, or even why drug use started climbing in the 1990s?

The well-intentioned effort to treat both legal and illegal substances the same has created other problems as well. For example, some elementary prevention materials identify marijuana, alcohol, heroin, and caffeine as drugs without making any distinctions among them. The children will soon realize that caffeine and alcohol are accepted and widely used in America. What does this do to their perception of the risk of marijuana, cocaine, or heroin? After all, they were each presented the same way. Consistent with this approach, one prevention specialist exuberantly described how a first-grade class responded to a prevention program by becoming very distressed about their parents' use of drugs. As the children left the program, many of them were crying. They all expressed commitment to talk their parents into giving up caffeine and alcohol. The prevention specialist thought it was wonderful. We wondered how many years it would take for these children to be embarrassed by what they had done. How will they then show that they are no longer "silly children"?

Another example is a poster showing a picture of a wine cooler with text stressing that wine coolers are drugs. The goal was to transfer a negative view of drugs to wine coolers, reducing their desirability. This could be a powerful prevention message for 5th graders. What happens, though, when the child becomes a high school senior and develops a positive view toward wine coolers? Could that acceptance generalize to "other" drugs? (I like wine coolers so maybe marijuana is not so bad.) After all, the child had years of prevention education emphasizing that alcohol is a drug, and that all drugs are virtually the same. While it may be technically correct to say, "A drug is a drug is a drug," there are serious, real-world differences between caffeine and cocaine, or even between wine coolers and heroin. Each drug carries its own risks, its own pharmacology, and its own cultural meanings. We cannot accurately treat drugs as one large category.

Young people are not the only ones who become confused by these over-simplified prevention messages. Parents who drink will not know how to cooperate with a message that labels them as drug users. Most prevention programs have not provided parents with any help in explaining this dichotomy to their children. *"Is alcohol a drug for children but not for adults? Why is it OK for adults but not for youth? If I want my children to abstain, do I have to give up alcohol? Is this a 'do as I say, not as I do' situation? What do I say? How do I say it?"* Many will opt to say nothing because they do not know what to say. Has youth-oriented prevention left parents out of prevention unless they abstain? That has not been the intent, but it has often been the reality. In fact, we sometimes have felt that the current prevention environment has created a whole new population of low-risk "closet drinkers" including parents, teachers, and prevention specialists!

Youth-focused prevention has also failed to prepare young people for the point in their own lives at which they can choose to drink legally. There may be vague references to the fact that someday they will be age 21 and allowed to drink, but prevention messages have left them completely unprepared for that day. They may be told that adults who drink should drink "responsibly," but that is never defined for them. Even aspirin comes with directions of how much to take and how often most people can use it without causing problems. However, alcohol does not come with directions. Neither does zero-tolerance, youth-focused prevention give any realistic guidance for drinking when a person reaches legal age.

Youth-focused prevention makes every decision only in terms of the teen and preteen years. The result has been prevention messages that are accepted by elementary or junior high students but rejected as the child moves toward high school and college age. Prevention must be capable of growing with a child and must involve meaningful adults in a child's life. At a minimum, this requires that we realistically address difficult issues such as what defines low-risk alcohol use, and why our society accepts low-risk drinking behavior for adults, but not for children. If prevention programs fail to help children make sense of this, the programs ultimately contribute to their own failure.

Making Nonuse a Youth Standard without Implying that Use Is the Adult Standard

Part of the nonuse strategy is to make abstinence the standard for young people. That is very reasonable. Yet, prevention messages do not occur in isolation. People receive and process these messages within their total experience of the culture. We must frame prevention messages within this larger context. There are at least two parts of our culture that are not being adequately addressed in the efforts to make nonuse a standard for youth. The first is specific to alcohol. Since the majority of adults drink, it would appear that *use* of alcohol is the standard for adults. With the national purchase age of 21, we have legally established drinking as an adult behavior. Taken as a whole, then, the message to young people is that abstaining is a child's behavior and drinking is an adult behavior. Teens are hungry to adopt adult behaviors. They are likely to adopt the opposite of any position or behavior they feel identifies them as a child. We have created an environment where drinking is an easy way for young people to separate themselves from childhood.

A second cultural context makes this situation even more difficult. In the United States, we simultaneously glorify youth while we encourage our children to adopt more and more adult behaviors. We have greatly extended the number of years before our children must take on *adult responsibilities* like self-sufficiency. At the same time, we give modern youth a great deal of *adult independence*. They largely decide the day-to-day course of their lives;

have significant amounts of expendable income; own their own cars; have their own jobs; and have many other freedoms and benefits of adult life. Why should we be surprised, then, when they adopt the few behaviors we have tried to keep exclusively adult—drinking and sex. If we allow our children more and more adult privileges, and treat them with adult independence, we should expect them to want to adopt these final "adult" behaviors.

We are not saying that drinking alcohol is mature or adult. Neither are we suggesting that adults should allow teens to drink. We are saying that youth-focused prevention has largely ignored adult drug and alcohol use while targeting children with slogans and laws aimed at keeping them from adopting these "adult" behaviors. Teens experience that prevention is for kids, not adults. The older teens get, the more they want to adopt the few adult "privileges" that they have not already adopted. Under these circumstances, any prevention success will be short-lived. Slogans and appeals to the law—especially when the law is not always backed up by action—have a short life. We cannot separate prevention from the larger context of our society. We cannot afford prevention approaches that focus on only one part of the lifespan as though the rest of it does not exist. Especially, we cannot afford to ignore adulthood and target *only* youth, while the larger environment is encouraging youth to act like adults.

Changing Our Focus

By focusing only on children and adolescents, prevention has failed to see and address several important variables. The zero-tolerance approach had enough strengths that, with a massive prevention campaign, it had some short-term positive impact. But it is just not possible to sustain that level of activity. America does not have the patience for a "100 year war" or even a "10 year war." Interest wanes. And when the flurry of funding and media attention dies down, the prevention effort must still be there, relevant and capable of meeting a broad range of needs for the whole population. We do not believe that youth-focused prevention has those capabilities.

We believe that a lifespan-focused approach can improve prevention and its effectiveness. At a minimum a lifespan-focused approach would meet three criteria. First, basic prevention concepts, definitions, and assumptions would be accurate and relevant throughout life. Second, prevention with youth would give young people clear and unambiguous expectations for their current behavior while simultaneously preparing them for their adult years. Third, we will conduct serious prevention efforts with adults as well as young people.

This implies that prevention programs will approach alcohol and illegal drugs somewhat differently. This is necessary to effectively address the fact that what is legal, socially acceptable, and low-risk changes over the lifespan. Currently available prevention models do not lend themselves to addressing these three issues. We need a lifespan-relevant prevention model.

HOW CAN A LIFESPAN-RELEVANT PREVENTION MODEL HELP?

Research-based prevention theory should play an important role in determining the direction of prevention activities. One aspect of prevention theory is developing models. People often use the word "model" to denote a program worth copying; however, this is not the way in which we are using the word. In this context, we are using "prevention model" to mean "a structured way of thinking that guides prevention programming." One could also use the word "paradigm." A prevention model provides the structured way of thinking that produces meaningful programs. Over the years, a variety of alcohol and drug models have evolved to guide prevention activities. The Prohibition Model was probably the first alcohol and drug prevention model. The Developmental Model became popular in the 1960s and 1970s. This model spawned affective education and curricula such as Magic Circle®, Quest®, Me-Me®, Omsbudsman®, and Project Charlie®. Also in the 1960s, the Normative Model led to responsible drinking and responsible decision-making approaches and curricula such as CASPAR® and

Here's Looking at You®. The Social Influences Model led to peer resistance education programs such as Project Smart®, Project Alert®, and DARE®. The Public Health Model provides an overall structure for prevention and has strongly influenced policy measures. More recently, the Risk and Resiliency Approach dramatically affected the direction of prevention, moving the field in a more generic direction. Hawkin's Social Development Model (Hawkins & Catalano, 1992) and Bernard's (1994) writings on resiliency are the most well-known sources of this approach.

Prevention Models Are Based on Assumptions of Cause

We further define a prevention model as "any structured way of thinking about prevention that contains two elements." First, a model gives one or more assumptions of causality—hopefully, but not always, research based. Second, a prevention model suggests strategies that logically flow from the causal assumptions. Thus, a prevention model will always articulate what causes the problem and logical steps to prevent the problem. For example, the Developmental Model is based on the belief that flaws in the developmental process cause drug problems. These flaws leave the person with low self-esteem, poor coping skills, poor decision-making skills, and poor communication skills. The suggested prevention is to raise self-esteem and increase personal and interpersonal skills. Affective education is the primary means used by the model to accomplish these goals. A 1960s articulation of the Normative Model (Plaut, 1967) suggested that alcohol problems were caused by a failure to normalize the presence of alcohol in society. This led to confusion, anxiety, and increased use. The strategy to prevent problems was to normalize alcohol use through responsible drinking education. The Prohibition Model is based on the belief that any use at all is likely to be harmful. The prevention strategy is to ban all alcohol or drug production and use. In general, one can take any prevention approach and work backward to find the assumption of cause. Together, the assumption of cause and the strategies to prevent form the prevention model.

If applied well, prevention models provide a coherency and consistency to prevention activities enhancing the likelihood of success. However, not all models will be successful. The history of prevention contains several examples of models that were logically developed and applied, but did not achieve the desired objectives. Yet, even the models that have provided poor results have added significantly to our knowledge of what works for whom, in what way, and under what circumstances.

Almost all popular prevention models currently in use seek to increase rates of nonuse among young people. Later in this monograph, we will review selected models in more detail, several of which have worked well for what they were designed to do. That is, these models were not designed to address the prevention needs of adults or to reduce high-risk use. Neither were they designed to assist young people in making the transition from adolescence to adulthood. This does not detract from their usefulness in helping to increase abstinence among young people. However, it does limit their application to lifetime prevention, leaving a serious void. A model that will fill this void must, at a minimum, provide a conceptual framework for addressing the three prevention goals cited earlier. These goals are: (1) increasing abstinence; (2) delaying the onset of use; and (3) reducing high-risk use. The new model also needs to recognize that what causes use and what causes problems are two different issues.

What Causes Use and What Causes Problems Are Different Questions

The failure to recognize the necessary questions has impeded development of lifetime-relevant prevention models. We have underscored the purpose of prevention as keeping problems from happening. Thus, when we talk about prevention models incorporating a statement of cause, we are referring to the cause of alcohol- and drug-related problems. *Unfortunately, it is not generally recognized that the questions (1) what causes alcohol and drug **problems**, and (2) what causes alcohol and drug **use** are two different questions with distinct answers.* Discussions of prevention theory often start out asking the first question and end up answering the second with no

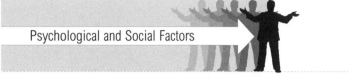

| Abstinence | Low-Risk Use | High-Risk Use | Problem Use | Alcoholism |

Figure 2.3. Alcoholism is not simply the end of a continuum of use.

apparent realization of the difference.[2] Certainly, complete success in preventing all use would prevent all use-related problems. But, as we have seen, prevention programs can achieve significant reductions in use without affecting related problems. The importance of reducing high-risk use for prevention has been largely overlooked because existing models have focused on the cause of use, rather than the cause of problems.

One assumption has been that any use causes problems, an assumption that is not well supported by research. Another assumption is that use and problems spring from the same source—also not well supported by research. This view treats all use as lying on a continuum that moves from "abstinence" to "moderate use" to "heavy use" to "problem use" to "addiction" (see Figure 2.3). In this view, the same forces act on the whole continuum of use. Thus, the only question is, "What causes use?" An unfortunate outcome of the continuum way of thinking is that it dismisses any role of use in causing problems, since the beginning of a continuum does not "cause" the end of a continuum. These ways of thinking view use and problems simply as results of the same psychosocial factors instead of recognizing that there are two separate questions.

In one of their early articles, Hawkins, Lishner, and Catalano (1985) began articulating the difference between the two questions: what causes problems, and what causes use. Hawkins noted that the prevention of experimentation (one form of use) and the prevention

---

[2] A good example of this is provided in the aforementioned first monograph published by the Office for Substance Abuse Prevention (now the Center for Substance Abuse Prevention; Dupont, 1989). The preface clearly identified the purpose—to "stop alcohol and drug *problems* before they occur." Yet the entire monograph focused on preventing *use*, with the apparent assumption that there is no difference in preventing use and preventing problems.

of drug abuse (one description of problem use) may require entirely different theories and approaches.[3] Unfortunately Hawkins did not develop the point further and the evolution of zero-tolerance prevention worked against addressing this difference. For example, we again call attention to the first monograph published by the Office for Substance Abuse Prevention (Dupont, 1989). Part of the philosophy presented by the committee was to *"not distinguish between 'use' and 'abuse' of drug chemicals (including alcohol and tobacco) by young people, but consider all such use to be abuse."* The U.S. Department of Education extended this point of view and published guidelines for selecting prevention materials that, among other things, advised against using any educational materials that distinguished between use and abuse. Both reports considered this distinction to be a "pro-drug" message. Both reports also warned against making any distinction between alcohol and illicit drugs in prevention messages.

If we make no distinction between substances, then we treat alcohol and illegal drugs the same. If we make no distinction between use and abuse, then we treat any use as being a problem. In either case, we are likely to ignore legitimate differences that exist between alcohol and illegal substances. We are equally unlikely to recognize legitimate differences between use that leads to problems and use that does not lead to problems (other than the use itself).

There are some very real and important distinctions between the two questions that could help make prevention programs more effective. Also, for both questions, there are differences between substances. For example, the psychological and social factors that are associated with low-risk alcohol use by adults and heroin use by teens are very different. The reasons for use are different, and the impact and outcomes are very different. Should the prevention

---

[3]Hawkins' specific statement (Hawkins, Lishner, & Catalano, 1985) is worth noting: "These considerations suggest that the prevention of *drug abuse* among adolescents may require a different strategy than the prevention of *experimentation* with drugs. Strategies which are adequate for preventing experimentation among those at low risk of engaging in serious antisocial behaviors may be wholly inadequate for preventing initiation and use by those who exhibit a 'deviance syndrome.' On the other hand, well-founded strategies for preventing drug abuse among those at highest risk for abuse may be inappropriate for those at risk only of becoming experimental users" (p. 78).

approach be the same? Research indicates (Newcomb & Bentler, 1988) that the psychosocial factors that correlate with the use of more socially acceptable substances are different from factors associated with less socially acceptable substances. Is it appropriate to assume that targeting prevention of alcohol use and crack use is the same for either teens or adults? For that matter, the factors associated with teenagers who drink no more than one beer twice a month and teenagers who get drunk twice a month are also very different. Should the prevention messages also be different? Research seems to clearly indicate (U.S. Department of Health and Human Services, 1996) that the majority of those who ever use alcohol, marijuana, or even cocaine never become dependent, or experience use-related problems. What are the differences among individuals who develop problems versus those who do not, and what are the implications for prevention?

Use is a prerequisite for dependence and other use-related problems, but use per se is not adequate to explain these problems. Thus, we must separately answer the questions of what causes drug problems and what causes drug use. Only then can we begin to understand why problems result for some people who use and not for others. This will provide a solid conceptual basis for developing programs that successfully increase the percentage who do not use drugs, and reduce problems among those who do use. Prevention theories and approaches that do not incorporate these differences cannot adequately address them.

There Are Multiple Categories of Use-Related Problems

The fact that alcohol and drug problems can be either health, impairment, or social problems further complicates the task of developing prevention models. Each of these categories can have different causes. Most use-related health problems occur from chronic high-risk use and can occur even if the user never becomes impaired. Impairment problems can occur with any occasion of high-risk use that causes impairment, even if the person does not use chronically. Social problems (such as arrests, family disapproval, work or school policy violations) can occur from any amount of use that is illegal, or socially unacceptable, even if it is neither chronic nor impairing. It is difficult to address all of these variables in a single model, but a model that successfully addresses the lifespan must do so.

There Is a Lifespan-Focused Model that Addresses These Issues

The next chapter introduces a specific model, the Lifestyle Risk Reduction Model. This model separately addresses the questions of what causes use and what causes problems associated with use. It also applies to all three types of use-related problems, and is useful for focusing our thinking and actions for *lifetime* prevention. The Lifestyle Risk Reduction Model, developed by Prevention Research Institute, Inc., is grounded in a health problems theory and applies to both impairment and social problems.

3

A Foundation for Lifespan-Focused Prevention

The constitutional tendency to this disease may be either inherited or acquired; but the disease is often induced by the habitual use of alcohol or other narcotic substances.

—Third Principle of the Society for the
Study and Cure of Inebriety, 1870

A comprehensive prevention model should apply to health problems, impairment problems, and social problems. In addition, prevention programs that address social or impairment problems should not contradict prevention efforts which target health problems. None should contradict recovery efforts. This is easy to articulate, but difficult to accomplish. For example, designated driver programs can reduce drunk driving but, by themselves, may contribute to continued high-risk drinking. The result may be other impairment problems or health problems. Also, the psychosocial theories that guide most prevention programs are typically designed to address social problems, and hardly refer to health problems. On the other hand, disease theory that guides most recovery programs starts with the assumption that alcohol and drug problems are health problems. Usually, disease theory ignores social problems, except as a symptom of alcohol or drug dependence. Consistent with these two approaches, several books proclaim addictions to be a disease (Milam & Ketcham, 1981),

49

while others proclaim addictions to be a lifestyle, or a "way of life" (Fingarette, 1988).

The Lifestyle Risk Reduction Model[1] addresses both prevention and recovery efforts for a lifetime. This model has characteristics of both a disease and a psychosocial model. More accurately, it is a bio-psycho-socio-behavioral model. The model explains the role played by each of these four factors and shows how the importance of each varies when we ask what causes the problem, versus what causes use. The nature and importance of each will also vary somewhat by type of problem—health, impairment, or social. By defining the role and relationship of these factors, a clearer picture emerges to guide prevention efforts. We will begin by applying the model to health problems.

Lifestyle-Related Health Problems

The Lifestyle Risk Reduction Model suggests that all alcohol- and drug-related health problems—including alcohol and drug dependence—are in the category of lifestyle-related health problems. As such, they share basic principles of both etiology and prevention with other lifestyle-related health problems, such as heart disease and many forms of cancer. Lifestyle-related health problems have a biological basis, but are triggered by lifestyle behaviors, rather than by a virus or bacteria.

There are two types of risk for lifestyle-related health problems. These could be broadly thought of as risks we can change and risks we cannot change. The risks we can change are some type of lifestyle behavior. This behavior always involves the quantity and frequency with which we experience such things as exercise, stress management, drug use, exposure to toxic chemicals, or dietary choices. The risks we cannot change are virtually always biological

---

[1] The Lifestyle Risk Reduction Model was articulated for the alcohol and drug field by Prevention Research Institute, Lexington, Kentucky, beginning in the late 1970s. Prevention Research Institute has published several research-based curricula that utilize this model. The five principles, five conditions, risk reduction formula, low-risk guidelines, and matrix that are presented were developed and copyrighted by Prevention Research Institute and are used by permission.

risks. These two types of risks interact in a simple formula: "Biological Risk + Quantity and Frequency Choices = Total Risk." Since we cannot control our biological risk, our only means of preventing lifestyle-related health problems is by adopting low-risk choices. The major role played by psychological and social factors is their influence on quantity and frequency choices.

Heart disease provides a readily understood example of lifestyle-related health problems. Most people accept that anyone can develop heart disease and that the basic nature of this risk is biological. Also, people with a family history of heart disease have greater biological risk. For example, research indicates that people who have a father, grandfather, or brother who died of heart disease before age 55 have a higher risk of developing heart disease. Similarly, having a mother, grandmother, or sister who died of heart disease before age 65 increases risk.

Thus, biological risk for heart disease is on a continuum. While anyone can develop heart disease, some people are more vulnerable than others. Biology establishes a "trigger level" at which the health problem will occur. People with a low level of biological risk have a high trigger level. That is, it will take longer for them to reach their trigger level and develop heart disease. People with increased biological risk have low trigger levels. Heart disease develops much more quickly and easily for these individuals. Between these two extremes lies a wide variety of risk levels and trigger levels (see Fig. 3.1).

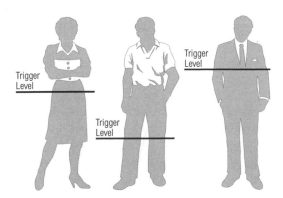

Figure 3.1. Different people have different "trigger levels."

If biology establishes a "trigger level" for heart disease, then lifestyle choices "pull the trigger." We are powerless over our level of biological risk, but not over our lifestyle choices. Quantity and frequency of fat intake, for example, will either increase or decrease risk. According to the American Heart Association, people who are more than 30 percent above their ideal weight are more likely to develop heart disease. By staying physically active, we cut our risk in half. On the other hand, if we choose to smoke, we double our risk for developing heart disease. Also, a reduction of 1 percent in blood cholesterol level reduces risk for heart disease by 2 percent. There is a variety of specific ways to reduce dietary fat. These include cooking with vegetable oil, limiting egg yolks to three or four per week, and limiting lean meat, fish, and poultry consumption to six ounces a day. The greater our level of biological risk, the more urgent the need for preventive behaviors which are all within our control.

However, we do not make our lifestyle choices in a vacuum. For example, with heart disease, personality traits such as hostility level and social norms around diet and exercise will influence choices and, thus, the rate of heart disease. In some places in the United States, eating traditional meals insures a high-fat diet. A person has to consciously work against these influences in order to achieve a low-fat diet. Factors such as social norms and personality do not cause heart disease, but they do influence our lifestyle choices.

In our experience, most Americans are familiar with the above understanding of heart disease. Most people know these preventive behaviors and many people practice them. From this understanding of heart disease, we would like to build a mental bridge to alcoholism. We will do this by applying the Five Principles of Lifestyle-Related Health Problems.

FIVE PRINCIPLES OF LIFESTYLE-RELATED HEALTH PROBLEMS

Principle One: Everyone Has Biological Risk

The first principle states that every person has an inborn level of biological risk (or vulnerability) for developing a health problem.

While everyone has some level of biological risk, different people have different levels of risk. When a high level of biological risk for any lifestyle-related health problem exists, it will typically show up in more than one family member.

Alcoholism frequently runs in families. However, most people receive both their genes and their family environment from the same parents. Thus, it is impossible for most family research to determine whether things pass from parent to child because of genes or family environment. However, adoption research allows us to examine the extent to which nature or nurture is most influential. This is possible because, in adoptees, one set of parents provides the genes while a different set of parents provides the family environment.

There have been three major adoption studies (Goodwin, 1984) completed for alcoholism. Each was completed since 1970—one in Denmark, one in the United States, and one in Sweden. Together these three independent studies include a sample of several thousand people and have remarkable consistency in their results. First, adoption research demonstrates that being raised with an adoptive parent who has alcoholism does not increase a child's risk for developing alcoholism. Adoptees whose biological parents did not have alcoholism all had the same rate of alcoholism as adults, regardless of whether they were raised with an alcoholic adoptive parent or nonalcoholic adoptive parents. Thus, adoption research indicates that alcoholism does not run in families because of the effect of living with an alcoholic parent. On the other hand, adoptees whose biological parent did have alcoholism, are four times (4×) more likely to develop alcoholism, even if raised by nonalcoholic adoptive parents. In other words, risk for alcoholism increased for those who had alcoholism in their biological parents, but not for those whose adoptive parents had alcoholism.

Other research (Schuckit, Goodwin, & Winokur, 1972) examined half-siblings who shared an alcoholic father, but were raised separately, one with the alcoholic father, the other not. As adults, they had the same rate of alcoholism. Being raised with the alcoholic parent did not increase risk for alcoholism, beyond the risk created by having a biological parent with alcoholism. Both adoption and the half-sibling research make it clear that increased risk for alcoholism runs in families because of increased biological risk, rather than from the effect of being raised with an alcoholic parent.

This is not to say that family environment does not influence children's drinking behavior; it does. One of the adoption studies found one aspect of family environment that was associated with increased risk for alcoholism. This characteristic, low socioeconomic status, had no direct link to alcoholism in the adoptive parent. The researchers noted that low socioeconomic status was also associated with heavy drinking in that culture (Cloninger, Bohman, & Sigvardsson, 1981). There are other ways that family environment can influence drinking behavior in the child. We will describe that impact later in this chapter. For now, we would note that the adoption research reported two overall findings that should not be broadened beyond their exact conclusions. First, being raised with an alcoholic parent *does not* increase risk for alcoholism as the child grows up. Second, having a biological parent with alcoholism *does* increase risk for alcoholism as the child grows up, even if the child is raised by nonalcoholic adoptive parents.

Twin research (Goodwin, 1984) also supports an important role for heredity in risk for alcoholism, as well as demonstrating the limits of heredity. Twin research (not adopted twins—just twins) is done by comparing concordance rates in identical, versus fraternal, twins. If a trait is the same in a twin pair, they are concordant; if not, they are discordant. The concordance rate is the percentage of time that both twins have the same feature or condition. There are three possibilities. The first is that the concordance rate is 100 percent in identical twins and less than 100 percent in fraternal twins, indicating that the condition being measured is genetically "controlled," since identical twins share 100 percent of their genes and fraternal twins share 50 percent, like any other siblings. For example, if one twin has blue eyes, the second will have blue eyes 100 percent of the time in identical twins, but not in fraternal twins. This indicates that eye color is genetically determined. The second possibility is that the concordance rate in identical twins is less than 100 percent, but is still higher than for fraternal twins. For example, the concordance rate for heart disease is less than 100 percent in identical twins, but is about twice as high as in fraternal twins. This indicates that heredity can increase risk for heart disease but, alone, does not determine whether heart disease will occur. The third possibility is that the concordance rate is less than 100 percent, but is the same in both identical and fraternal twins. This indicates that heredity plays no special role in the condition. An example of this could be whether the twins grew up in an apartment or a house.

Twin research on alcoholism has shown that the concordance rate for identical twins is well below 100 percent. This tells us that, like heart disease, heredity can predispose a person to alcoholism, but does not predestine its development. However, research shows that if one identical twin develops alcoholism, the chances that the second twin will develop alcoholism are about twice as high as those for fraternal twins. Together, these findings tell us that heredity plays an important role in establishing risk for alcoholism, but heredity does not act alone (Murray, Clifford, & Gurling, 1983).

Once research established that children of alcoholics had increased biological risk for alcoholism, the next step was to compare their biological response to alcohol to that of children of nonalcoholics. An interesting series of studies being done by Schuckit and Smith (1996) is providing more specific information about biological risk for alcoholism. The research is being conducted with a group of men identified as having either a family history of alcoholism or no family history of alcoholism.[2] The study began when the men were college age and only included those who were not showing any signs of alcohol problems. One of the very early findings that distinguished the two groups was that those with a family history of alcoholism were four times more likely to have a high tolerance to alcohol.[3] That is, it took more alcohol for them to show signs of

[2]Women have now been added to the study as well, but no data are available at this time.

[3]Schuckit uses the term "low sensitivity" to mean that, at the blood alcohol levels measured, these people became less impaired than is typical of most people. Sensitivity, or initial tolerance, refers to the initial or inborn level of impairment that a person has to a given blood alcohol level. People who from the beginning of their drinking experience can "drink other people under the table" would have a low sensitivity or a high initial tolerance. Acquired tolerance, often simply referred to as tolerance, refers to an increase in the blood alcohol level needed to cause impairment. Schuckit measured both sensitivity (initial tolerance) and acquired tolerance. Since most people are familiar with the concept of tolerance, but few people understand the concept of sensitivity to alcohol, we have chosen to use the phrase "high tolerance," to refer to what Schuckit called low sensitivity.

intoxication. Could this finding help explain the increased risk for alcoholism demonstrated by adoption studies for biological children of alcoholics? The answer appears to be "yes."

Over a nine-year follow-up period, Schuckit's data showed that having a family history of alcoholism and demonstrating high tolerance (or low sensitivity) to alcohol were independent risk factors for developing alcoholism. Similar to the adoption research, Schuckit found that children of alcoholics, irrespective of tolerance, had almost three times an increased risk for developing alcoholism over the nine-year follow-up period. When looking only at high tolerance, without taking into account family history, those with a high tolerance were four times more likely to develop alcoholism compared to those with a low tolerance. Thus, both family history of alcoholism and high tolerance increased risk for developing alcoholism with high tolerance appearing to be the stronger predictor. But the combination effect was even more potent. Specifically, about 15 percent of the children of alcoholics who did *not* have high tolerance to alcohol in their early twenties qualified for a *Diagnostic and Statistical Manual of Mental Disorders Third Edition* (DSM-III) alcohol diagnosis over the nine years. But among those who had a family history of alcoholism and a high tolerance, 60 percent qualified for a DSM-III diagnosis of either alcohol abuse or alcohol dependence within the nine year follow-up!

This research suggests that there are at least two identifiable indicators of increased biological risk for alcoholism: family history and high tolerance. As with heart disease, prevention practitioners could help people learn about their probable level of biological risk by asking questions about family history. The predictive value of high tolerance to alcohol suggests the importance of also asking questions about tolerance levels. Together, these two biological risk indicators provide the most powerful predictor of risk for developing alcoholism currently available.

The data on biological risk is as relevant for alcoholism as for heart disease. Both alcoholism and heart disease demonstrate the first principle of lifestyle-related health problems: Biology establishes a level of risk for the condition, and that level of risk varies from person to person. We cannot control our biological risk, but knowledge of that risk provides important information for our behaviors.

Principle Two: The Quantity and Frequency of Specific Choices Create Risk

For every lifestyle-related health problem, there is some behavior that creates risk. Sometimes the only low-risk choice is to abstain completely from that behavior. In most cases, however, there is a threshold of risk. Any amount above that threshold is high risk and any amount below is low risk. For skin cancer, the behavior is exposure to the sun. For lung cancer, it is smoking. For heart disease, it is diet and exercise. The behavioral counterpart for alcoholism and other alcohol-related problems is the quantity and frequency of drinking. Unlike heart disease, however, few of us have been taught which specific behaviors are low risk for developing alcoholism or other alcohol-related problems. To the best of our knowledge, alcohol, caffeine, and tobacco are the only legal drugs that do not come with guidance about the levels of consumption that are not likely to cause problems. Aspirin, antihistamines, and other legal drugs come with specific guidelines about what constitutes low-risk use. The need to provide this information for medications is apparent but seems to have been overlooked when it comes to alcohol.

Instead, alcohol prevention messages have focused either on not drinking at all, or on drinking "moderately" or "responsibly." While total abstinence works completely for those who choose it, only 30 percent to 40 percent of the drinking age population in the United States currently makes that choice. Prevention programs admonish the 70 percent who drink to drink moderately or responsibly. However, these terms are rarely defined in a practical way. What does it mean to drink moderately? How does a person know when drinking is responsible? Some suggest that outcome is the best way to measure responsible drinking (Plaut, 1967). The problem with this approach is that if a person waits until a problem occurs to know that the drinking was irresponsible, it is too late for prevention. Effective prevention allows a person to be able to assess risk ahead of time and to know what behaviors reduce risk.

When we see alcohol-related problems as lifestyle-related problems, the need for specifically defined low-risk choices becomes obvious. The guidelines, though, would need to take into account both health and impairment problems with special guidance for avoidance of the social problems that do not involve quantity and frequency of consumption. We will propose such guidelines under the Five Conditions of Risk Reduction in Chapter 5.

Principle Three: The Level of Biological Risk Determines the Quantity and Frequency that Will Be High Risk

Since our quantity/frequency choices interact with our biology, it makes sense that the higher the level of biological risk, the fewer high-risk choices it will take to trigger a health problem. We cannot control our level of biological risk. However, knowing our level of biological risk will provide critical information about the importance of our choices. It will also tell us exactly what behaviors will be low risk for us.

Family history is one way to measure biological risk for alcoholism. The greater the number of blood relatives with alcoholism, the closer they are in the bloodline, and the younger they were when the alcoholism developed, the greater the risk is for alcoholism. For example, among people who develop alcoholism, those with a family history of alcoholism develop alcoholism 10 years earlier than those who do not have a family history (Goodwin, 1984). One study (McKenna & Pickens, 1981) compared the length of time between first drink and first intoxication episode and between first intoxication and apparent onset of alcoholism. It compared a group of patients based on whether neither parent, one parent, or both parents had alcoholism. The relationship was linear. Those with no alcoholic parents averaged the longest time between the three episodes, those with two alcoholic parents averaged the shortest time, and those with one alcoholic parent fell in the middle. In this case, time directly corresponds to quantity and frequency of drinking. For those with two alcoholic parents, it took less drinking to develop alcoholism. For those with nonalcoholic parents, it took more drinking to develop alcoholism.

As indicated earlier, alcohol response is also an important measure of biological risk. Those who are born with, or acquire, a high tolerance (low sensitivity) to alcohol have significantly greater risk. Those who have a family history of alcoholism and a high tolerance have the greatest risk. Thus, the amount of drinking that would be low risk for these different groups would vary depending on their individual levels of biological risk.

Principle Four: Health Problems Occur when the Level of High-Risk Choices "Matches" the Level of Biological Risk

This principle illustrates the interaction in the core part of the formula. Biology alone cannot cause the health problem. Neither can quantity and frequency alone cause a health problem. It is only in combination that the lifestyle-related health problem emerges.

People commonly assume that the kind of person we are determines whether or not we will develop alcoholism. Alcoholism is widely viewed as occurring only, or primarily, in those people who are either emotionally troubled or "weak willed." Prevention programs inadvertently encourage this view by labeling attributes such as low self-esteem as the primary cause of alcohol and drug problems. But the very act of identifying something specific as the cause implies that other factors are not the cause. If alcoholism occurs because of the kind of person I am then the implication is that I do not have to worry about my drinking choices. I only have to avoid being "that kind of person."

While many people believe that an abnormal, prealcoholic personality determines who will develop alcoholism, research has failed to identify one. Several personality traits have been identified as encouraging high-risk drinking or drug-taking behavior, but in no way would these behaviors appear to be limited to any form of emotional pathology. Most personality traits and emotional problems that are so common among people who have alcoholism appear to develop over the course of the addiction and seem to be emotional consequences of drinking rather than causes. Barnes (1979) has identified these as making up the "clinical alcoholic personality." With a few exceptions that we will note later, it seems appropriate to conclude that alcoholism is found in both emotionally healthy and

unhealthy people. Both psychologically and biologically, then, anyone can develop alcoholism.

Research supports the fourth principle. In the case of addiction
or any other alcohol-related health problem, the most direct cause
is simply the interaction of an individual's level of biological risk
combined with the quantity and frequency of alcohol intake. When
the level of high-risk drinking matches the level of biological risk,
addiction develops. We will indicate how this principle applies to
impairment problems and social problems later.

This is not to say that alcohol consumption can be used to
diagnose alcoholism any more than fat intake can be used to diagnose heart disease. Rather, quantity of drinking combined with
inborn biological risk triggers alcoholism.

From a prevention perspective, both parts of this equation
are important. First, understanding the formula can help move
people away from the false belief that the kind of person they are
will protect them. Once that is understood, people can see that
while they cannot change their biology, they can estimate their
biological risk. Behavior is the most important part of the prevention equation since it is the only part of the formula that is within
a person's control.

The fourth principle presents an interesting challenge for preventing alcoholism and other alcohol-related problems. We must help
people understand that preventing problems has little to do with the
kind of person they are and everything to do with the kind of choices
they make. Thus, we need to help people reduce high-risk choices
and increase abstinence and other low-risk choices. How to accomplish that is the focus of the rest of this book. The fifth principle
begins to point the way.

Principle Five: Social and Psychological
Factors Influence Quantity and
Frequency Choices

The fifth principle adds two arrows to the formula that we gave
earlier. One arrow comes from psychological factors and the other
from social factors. Both go to the quantity and frequency choices

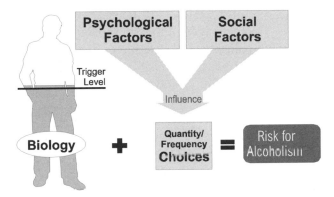

Figure 3.2.   The Lifestyle Risk Reduction formula.

(see Fig. 3.2). The basic part of the formula, "biology + quantity/ frequency," answers the question, "What causes problems?" The arrows address the question, "What causes use?"

Psychological Influences

There is wide agreement that psychological factors are important in the development of alcoholism. However, there is wide disagreement on exactly which factors are important and what role they play. For example, evidence shows (Barnes, 1979; Levenson et al., 1990) that personality traits such as high sensation–seeking (or novelty-seeking), rebelliousness, gregariousness, and impulsiveness influence drinking behaviors. People sometimes assume that psychological factors directly cause alcoholism; yet, there does not appear to be anything about these traits that directly causes alcoholism. It is easy to imagine, though, how these traits influence a person toward high-risk drinking.

Attitudes are another psychological influence. There has been debate in the psychology literature as to whether attitudes influence behavior. We maintain that attitudes are significant influences on drinking behavior and that this can be demonstrated if certain attitudes are measured. We believe that one of the problems with research in this area is that attitudes are treated as though they are a single entity. Any sampling of attitudes about drinking is treated as a reasonable measure of the role of attitudes. Our own experience does not support this. In an attempt to better understand the role of attitudes in drinking behavior, the first author and a colleague, Dr. Merita Thompson, examined over 120 attitude statements in the late 1970s. Less than 20 of these statements were strongly related to drinking behavior. After further refinement, Prevention Research Institute designed curricula to alter these attitudes and related behaviors in several different audiences (Daugherty & O'Bryan, 1986). Thompson and Costello (Thompson, 1996) evaluated the curriculum designed for college students and found that there were statistically significant changes in both attitudes and behaviors. Their evaluation also demonstrated that attitude and behavior changes in the experimental group occurred concurrently in the predicted direction (p = .0001). The smaller fluctuations that occurred in the control group were random. Further support came from the Iowa Alcohol Research Consortium evaluation (Engen, Richards, & Patterson, 1995) of Prevention Research Institute's curriculum for drunk driving offenders (Daugherty & O'Bryan, 1986). This study demonstrated that changes in these same attitudes at post-test were predictive of nonrecidivism over a three-year period. In these evaluations and others (Marsteller, Falek, & Rolka, 1997), one strong predictor was the attitude that getting drunk was a good way to have fun. Other strong predictors were attitudes relating to whether the person viewed alcohol problems as primarily resulting from drinking or from personal weakness. Conversely, people who believed they could avoid problems through personal strength were more likely to continue making high-risk choices.

There is also the question of whether alcoholism is a manifestation of underlying psychopathology. McCord and McCord's (1960) longitudinal study of inner-city children indicated that childhood behavioral problems predicted later alcoholism as adults. This study is frequently cited to support the view that alcoholism is caused by underlying pathology. However, the study is limited because it did not control for family history of alcoholism and the sample was drawn from a clinical population. Another study that better addresses this question is Vaillant's (1995) 50-year longitudinal natural history study. Vaillant included both a college sample and an inner-city sample, neither of which were clinical populations.

This natural history study found no evidence that psychopathology preceded alcoholism. Most of those who developed alcoholism were notably free of preexisting pathology or family dysfunction.

There is no dispute that, at the point of contact with the treatment system, people with alcoholism typically exhibit psychopathology. However, we need to ask three questions. First, "Is the rate of dysfunction among people with alcoholism as high for those who do not seek treatment as among those who do?" The answer is "no" (Regier et al., 1990). Those who seek treatment are a self-selected group who are the most desperate and least functional. The group that does not seek treatment appears to have less pathology. Thus, people in treatment for alcoholism are not a representative sample.

Second, "Is the rate of dysfunction higher among those with alcoholism than it is in the general population?" The answer is "yes" (Regier et al., 1990), but that is meaningless until we answer a third question which is, "Does a careful history reveal that the drinking typically precedes the emotional dysfunction, or that the dysfunction typically precedes the drinking?" Clearly both occur in different situations. There are at least two relatively large studies and several small studies that address this question (Schuckit & Hesselbrock, 1994; Schuckit, Irwin, & Brown, 1990). In the larger studies, there is some indication that anxiety disorders may often precede alcoholism. However, the smaller, better controlled studies indicate that when anxiety disorders and depression coexist with alcoholism, the alcoholism most typically develops first. The fact that depression and anxiety disorders frequently (though not always) clear up without treatment once the person abstains further indicates that often they are a result of alcoholism.

There is agreement in the research literature (Hesselbrock et al., 1984) that antisocial personality disorder does occur more frequently among those with alcoholism and that, when it occurs, it typically precedes, or at least mutually coexists with, the alcoholism. This disorder occurs in about 16 percent to 20 percent of those with alcoholism. There is reason to believe that, like alcoholism, heredity can play a role in development of antisocial personality disorder, and that genetic risk for the two conditions can overlap. In the largest adoption study, Cloninger et al. (1981) identified two patterns of alcoholism that they referred to as Type 1 and Type 2.

Type 2 alcoholism is characterized by early onset and antisocial or criminal behavior. The hereditary link appeared to be father to son and, if the father presented this type of alcoholism, the risk that the son would develop it was increased nine times. It appears that this type of alcoholism represents an overlap of alcoholism and antisocial personality disorder, and that the combined genetic influence may account for the very high level of increased risk.

A smaller adoption study in the United States, by Cadoret and Gath (1978), supported a similar conclusion. This study found two factors that predicted adult alcoholism among the adoptees. One was having a biological parent with alcoholism, and the other was presence of childhood conduct disorder. Conduct disorder is the childhood diagnosis that often precedes an antisocial personality disorder diagnosis among adults. Unfortunately, Cadoret's finding is sometimes used to support a position that childhood conduct disorder is independently predictive of alcoholism, and that alcoholism is a result of underlying psychopathology. However, in a personal conversation with Cadoret in 1980, he stated that, among the adoptees who had childhood conduct disorder and then developed alcoholism as adults, 100 percent also had a biological parent with alcoholism. He further noted that the adoptive parents believed that the disruptive behavior occurred prior to any drinking. However, the adoptees themselves reported that they were drinking prior to the occurrence of the behavior problems, but that their parents were unaware of their drinking.

At this point in time, the literature supports the conclusion that increased genetic risk for alcoholism and increased risk for antisocial personality disorder often occur in the same families. But antisocial personality disorder may not be the only behavioral problem that correlates with alcoholism and is a result of being the child of an alcoholic. Several studies (Sher, 1994; Tarter, Hegedus, Goldstein, Shelly, & Alterman, 1984; Whipple, Parker, & Noble, 1988) have found that attention deficit disorder and a variety of cognitive, neurological difficulties are more common among those with alcoholism and their children. It appears to be most accurate to consider attention deficit disorder and other neurological differences as often accompanying alcoholism, rather than a psychological "causes" of alcoholism.

Clearly, psychological factors play a role in the development of alcoholism and, thus, will be important in both prevention and recovery. The question is, "What is the nature of that role?" The Lifestyle Risk Reduction Model suggests that the role played by psychological factors is one of influencing quantity/frequency choices rather than directly causing alcoholism. This is true whether we are talking about personality traits, attitudes, or those occasions when a psychological problem precedes alcoholism. Psychological factors help answer the question, "What causes use?"

Social Influences

Research has consistently demonstrated a powerful role for social factors in influencing drinking and drug-taking behaviors. The importance of cultural norms in influencing both drinking behavior and rates of alcoholism has been clear since the 1940s. Bales (1944) published a landmark study indicating that different rates of alcoholism in different groups could be explained by cultural factors. More recently, social research has demonstrated the important role that laws on taxation and sales restrictions can have on reducing consumption (West, 1984).

Religion also has a very significant influence on drinking behavior. Numerous studies (Cahalan & Room, 1974; Clark & Hilton, 1991) indicate that those who are involved in religious activities tend to drink less than those who have no religious affiliation. There are also differences within religious affiliations. Members of religious groups who hold an abstinence position abstain at significantly higher rates than other religious groups. However, there is some indication that they may also have higher rates of heavy drinking among those who are affiliated, but not involved. It appears that young people who attend religious services as few as five times a year drink less (Schlegel & Sanborn, 1979). It is also interesting that there is less drinking among adolescents who attend services regularly, but whose parents do not, than there is among those whose parents attend with them (Burkett, 1977). This does not mean that it is best for parents not to attend religious services with their children. Rather, it seems likely that teenagers who attend church regularly, in spite of no parental involvement, have a high degree of commitment to their religious beliefs.

The drinking behavior of friends and family correlates strongly with drinking for both adolescents (Hawkins, Lishner, & Catalano, 1985) and adults (Harburg, DiFranceisco, Webster, Gleiberman, & Schork, 1990). In fact, the role of family in influencing drinking behavior is so well established and deeply rooted that many people have difficulty accepting the adoption research. But the two bodies of research are not in conflict. Adoption research clearly indicates that alcoholism runs in families, more because of heredity than the effect of being raised with a parent who has alcoholism. But this does not imply that parental drinking does not influence the drinking behavior of children.

In fact, evidence from a variety of sources (Cisin & Cahalan, 1968; Goodwin, 1984) shows that children of alcoholics who are raised by an alcoholic parent actually have a somewhat higher rate of abstaining. As a result, they have a lower risk for developing alcoholism than those who are raised separately from an alcoholic parent. If this seems counterintuitive, it is helpful to recognize that a parent's behavior may influence a child positively or negatively. A child may adopt the parent's behavior or be repelled by it and avoid the behavior. At least one study found that children of heavy drinkers are more likely to also drink heavily if they are unaware of problems associated with the parents' drinking. However, among those who are aware of problems associated with the parents' drinking, the rates of abstinence or minimal drinking will be higher. (Harburg et al., 1990). This is consistent with general population surveys (Cisin & Cahalan, 1968) that have shown higher rates of abstinence among those who have a close relative with alcoholism. Other studies (Pandina & Johnson, 1990) indicate that overall rates of heavy drinking are no higher among children of alcoholics through high school and college age. Together, this body of research indicates that families affect risk for alcoholism primarily through heredity but affect abstaining primarily through social influence.

Other evidence that parents can influence the alcohol and drug behaviors of their children comes from prevention research. The Addiction Research Foundation (Shain, Suurvali, & Kilty, 1980) conducted one of the earliest evaluations on parent education as a prevention strategy. They examined the impact of a Canadian program based on Parent Effectiveness Training. Following a Developmental Model, the hypothesis was that by improving communication and the relationship between parent and child, the likelihood of alcohol or drug use by the children would decrease. The program was successful in increasing parent/child communication and bonding, but the outcomes related to use failed to support the hypothesis. Instead they found that the improved parent/child relationship increased the chances the child would adopt the parent's alcohol and drug behaviors. Thus, if the parent drank, the child was more likely to drink. If the parent abstained, the child was more likely to abstain. This study clarified that bonding does not increase the likelihood of abstinence. It increases the likelihood that the child will adopt the parent's behaviors.

Prevention Research Institute took another approach to parent education in 1983 using a curriculum based on the Lifestyle Risk Reduction Model. The curriculum is designed to modify parents' high-risk drinking and prepare parents to communicate both risk-reduction information and clear behavioral expectations to their children. A one-year controlled study by Van Tubergen, Daugherty, O'Bryan, and Morrow (Thompson, 1996) indicated a reduction in high-risk drinking by the parents as well as an increase in abstinence and decrease in high-risk drinking by the teens. This also illustrates that parents can influence the drinking behavior of their children.

Like psychological factors, there is no doubt that social factors play an important role in the etiology of drinking behaviors and of alcoholism, but it is important to identify the specific role that they play. The Lifestyle Risk Reduction Model stresses that norms, friends, family, religion, and other social influences do not directly cause alcoholism any more than they directly cause heart disease; but, social factors do influence whether a person drinks high-risk or low-risk quantities.

Putting It All Together

Imagine Sue, whose mother and grandfather had alcoholism at a young age. Sue has always been able to drink almost everyone "under the table," an ability of which she is quite proud. She has always been a high sensation–seeking person who loves to try new things. She is also a gregarious person who loves to be with groups to party. In addition, she has always felt that rules applied to other people, if they were rigid enough to be bound by rules. She established a successful business and is very confident in her ability to handle whatever life brings her.

Sue loves to drink, and usually drinks quite a bit. Is it likely that at tonight's party, Sue will have one glass of wine and enjoy the evening visiting with friends? It certainly is possible. But, it seems more likely that she will drink the whole bottle of wine and hardly feel impaired. Are psychological and social influences playing a significant role in this impending case of alcoholism? Absolutely. They influence her high-risk choices. What is going to cause her to develop alcoholism? It is the interaction of the quantity and frequency of high-risk drinking with her level of biological risk.

The most effective prevention program would address all of those factors. She will need to understand that she is not protected by her high self-esteem, her high tolerance, or her success. She needs to understand the formula—what is in her control and what is not. She also needs to understand how the psychological and social influences in her life are propelling her toward alcoholism. Finally, she needs support in changing her behavior and discovering psychological and social support for the new behavior. We will address this further in Chapter 5.

How Does the Formula Address Impairment and Social Problems?

While health problems take months or years of high-risk drinking to develop, impairment problems can occur in one occasion of high-risk use. We define impairment problems as acute problems that occur as a result of alcohol- or drug-induced impairment in physical or mental functioning. This includes problems such as impaired driving, fights, falls, or poor job/school performance. With one adjustment, the Lifestyle Risk Reduction formula can be applied to impairment problems. The basic part of the formula remains: Biology + Quantity/Frequency. When referring to impairment problems, however, biology does not refer to the trigger level, or the point at which a health problem will occur. Instead, it refers to the tolerance level—the point at which impairment will occur. When a person drinks enough to reach his tolerance level, impairment occurs. Then any situation that involves risk can lead to impairment problems.

With impairment problems, the psychological and social factors influence not only the quantity/frequency choices but also the situations in which people find themselves and their behavior in those situations. As a result, impairment problems are less tied to quantity and frequency than to health problems. For example, those who have rebellious personalities are more likely to put themselves in situations where impairment will lead to problems. They are also more likely to violate laws or get in fights. Similarly, low self-esteem has not been associated with increased drinking (Schroeder, Laflin, & Weis, 1993) but has been associated with increased problems related to use (Walitzer & Sher, 1996). Once again, it seems likely that those with low self-esteem may be more likely to put themselves in harm's way when they drink. It also should come as no surprise that alcohol-related health problems are more common among the affluent, while impairment and social problems are more common among those of low socioeconomic status. The affluent drink more because they can afford it and are frequently in heavy drinking situations. Again, health problems are more a function of quantity and frequency plus biology. But the affluent can insulate themselves somewhat from many impairment and social problems. They are less likely to be drinking on the street, more likely to have cab fare, more likely to be drinking at home, in the safety of a friend's home, or in a private club. The police may be more likely to excuse their behavior and escort them home.

Some social problems occur as a result of any use, not as a result of either impairment or any other high-risk use. These may include occasions when any use is illegal or a violation of work or school policy. It could also include a violation of parental or family expectations, a violation of seriously held social norms or religious beliefs, or any behavior that is otherwise socially inappropriate. This includes adolescent alcohol use, illicit drug use, or drinking on the job. In this case, the formula does not exactly apply, since such social problems do not result from an interaction of biology and quantity/frequency. It is, however, still a quantity/frequency issue, with the appropriate quantity and frequency being zero. The interaction in this situation is with social factors, not with biology.

Although the interaction of the variables in the formula is more complex for impairment problems and certain social problems, the prevention issue is still the same. The variable that we can best individually control and most productively target for prevention is quantity/frequency. As already noted, alcohol and drug prevention programs have tended to focus on use without regard to quantity/frequency, or have focused on preventing impairment problems through measures such as using designated drivers. It is difficult to argue with the logic that impaired drivers should use designated drivers. In our opinion, there is a place for designated drivers in comprehensive prevention strategies. But designated drivers enable designated drinkers to continue making high-risk drinking choices. The driving problem may have been averted, but the family, job, or health problem may have been encouraged. Only by reducing high-risk choices can we reduce all use-related problems.

SUMMARY

The Lifestyle Risk Reduction Model presents alcohol- and drug-related health problems—including addiction—as being in the category of lifestyle-related health problems. Thus, they share basic principles with other lifestyle-related health problems such as heart disease and many forms of cancer. Lifestyle-related health problems are those in which there is a biologically established level of risk and in which lifestyle choices serve as the triggering agent. Examples of such lifestyle choices include exposure to the sun for skin cancer, exposure to cigarette smoke for lung cancer, amount of exercise and dietary fat for heart disease, and consumption of alcohol for alcoholism. The level of biological risk determines the quantity and frequency of the given lifestyle choices that are likely to trigger a problem. Psychosocial factors are most important in etiology and prevention by influencing the quantity/frequency choices.

4

Learning from Youth-Focused
Prevention Models

A hundred times every day I remind myself that my inner
and outer lives are based on the labors of other men,
living and dead, and that I must exert myself in order to
give in the same measure as I have received and am still
receiving.

—Albert Einstein

We have stated that it is necessary to move beyond youth-focused
prevention and embrace the lifespan. We do not want that to imply,
however, that youth-focused prevention has nothing to offer. On the
contrary, the models guiding youth-focused prevention have made
important contributions to our understanding of effective prevention
programming, especially with youth. As is often the case, learning
comes from both success and failure. In this chapter, we present four
influential youth-focused prevention models. Our intention is to
identify lessons learned and describe how to integrate these models
into a Lifestyle Risk Reduction approach.

AFFECTIVE DEVELOPMENT

The first youth-focused model evolved at least two decades
before youth-focused prevention became the dominant prevention

mode. The Affective Development Model is also referred to as affective education. It proposes that alcohol and drug use results from flaws in the developmental process. This results in low self-esteem, poor communication skills, poor problem-solving and coping skills, and poor decision-making skills. This model has also been called the "Deficiencies Model" (Falck & Craig, 1988). Affective education focuses on feelings and values clarification rather than skill development. The skill development focuses on intrapersonal skills, rather than interpersonal, and is usually general rather than alcohol or drug specific. Thus, teaching decision-making skills focuses on the internal decision-making process. Any practice or application may be with situations that do not involve alcohol or drugs. The model assumes that once the skill is learned, it will be applied to alcohol and drugs and will withstand peer pressures. Similarly, students may learn assertiveness skills without these skills specifically applied to alcohol and drugs. Affective education, then, was the first of the "generic" prevention approaches. Generic prevention refers to prevention that focuses on general skill development rather than a specific problem. It promises to positively impact a variety of problems such as alcohol and drug use, juvenile delinquency, adolescent pregnancy, and/or violence.[1]

Initially, affective education focused on grades 1–3. It used activities designed to help children recognize and understand their emotions, bond to their classes and teachers, feel good about themselves, problem solve, learn decision-making, and develop coping skills. The most popular of these early programs were Magic Circle® and Tribes®. Later, affective education was expanded to grades 4–6 and then to 7–8 with programs like: Project Charlie®, Here's Looking at You 1 & 2®, Me-Me®, and Omsbudsman®. Finally, affective education was extended to older grades with programs like Quest®. The impact of the affective education approach went far beyond the curricula. Perhaps its biggest success was in convincing many

---

[1] The term "generic prevention" has also been applied to prevention that *includes* both alcohol and drugs, but is not *specific* to a particular substance such as alcohol, tobacco, or marijuana. When used in this way, the term does not imply inclusion of such things as violence or juvenile delinquency. For example, Tobler and Stratton used the word in this way in their 1997 report on meta-analysis. As with most terms, it is useful to clarify how the word is being used.

professionals and the general public that low self-esteem was the basis for most youth problems. Research only lends minimal support to this assumption. The primary support for affective education is the belief that people hold in it.

The impact of affective education appears to be limited. Several reviews of affective education (Falck & Craig, 1988; Hansen, 1990; Tobler & Stratton, 1997) have indicated no impact on alcohol or drug use. Hansen's (1990) review of research on affective education was probably the most positive, showing that about one-third of the studies had no impact, another third showed some positive impact, and the remainder showed a negative impact on alcohol and drug use.

SOCIAL INFLUENCES MODEL

While affective education focuses on internal and personal shortcomings as causes of drug use, the Social Influences Model focuses on external factors. The Social Influences Model was first applied successfully to cigarette smoking and, later, to alcohol and marijuana use. The model is based on the assumption that initiation of drug use most commonly results from social pressures that the young person is not prepared to withstand. The model does not assume that "pro-use" attitudes precede initial drug use. Instead, the model holds that first use usually occurs at a time when the young person still holds antiuse attitudes. However, if not prepared for social pressure, the young person may succumb to use. The use itself then may alter attitudes in a way that supports continued use.

Programs based on this model include Project Smart[8], Project Alert[8], STAR[8], and DARE[8]. To prevent first use, these programs focus on young people at a time when they tend to hold negative attitudes toward use—usually in the 5th or 6th grade. They use a variety of strategies including peer resistance training, correcting misperceptions of the norm, and inoculating against mass media messages. They also assist in dealing with family influences to use, give information about consequences of use, and ask for public commitments to nonuse. Peer leaders usually facilitate the peer resistance lessons and build support for nonuse.

    Each of these programs use peer resistance training to teach
students a variety of ways to resist pressure or opportunities to use
alcohol and drugs. Evaluations indicate that in order to be effective,
peer resistance lessons need to be facilitated by peers and actively
involve students in multiple practice sessions. Teaching the skills on
video or without follow-up practice sessions has not been as successful. Project Smart® used a sociogram technique that allowed
each classroom of students to identify a student in the class whom
they would like to teach them the skills. Sometimes the students
chosen as peer leaders were gang members or other "tough kid"
types. This approach may be superior to the traditional approach to
peer leadership in which adults choose peer leaders. Adults often
choose young people that they favor but whom the students may not
consider a credible source of information.

    Techniques to correct misperceptions of the norm are a key part
of Project Smart®, Project Alert®, and STAR®. These techniques
grew out of findings that most young people believe use is more
accepted and more common than is actually true. To overcome these
misperceptions, programs sometimes make comparisons to national
or local use data. Other times, programs use classroom surveys that
allow students to experience the misperceptions within their own
peer group. This simple and effective technique has the benefit of
immediate and personal feedback. Anonymous surveys ask for a
person's own response as well as how they think the rest of the group
will respond. For example, one of the statements could be, "It is OK
to get drunk." If there are 25 children in the class, a student might
respond "I strongly disagree." "Of the remaining 24 in my class I
think 3 others will strongly disagree, 6 will disagree, 5 will agree,
and 10 will strongly agree." Much to the students' surprise, there is
usually less support for use and less use happening than believed.
For example, when the anonymous responses are tallied for all
questions, the student might discover that 12 strongly disagreed and
6 disagreed while only 4 agreed and 2 strongly agreed. Studies
indicate that this simple process can reduce use. It is an excellent
example of how "peer pressure" can have nothing to do with one
person pressuring another, and more to do with people pressuring
themselves to do what they think their peers are expecting. This
technique can "relieve" some of that mistaken peer pressure. A

variety of studies reported that activities designed to correct misperceptions of the norm can help bring about behavior change, perhaps even with young adults. In fact, one Project Smart® researcher (Hansen, 1990) reported that changing misperceptions of the norm was the most important activity in the program.

Both the media and the family messages in this approach are designed to help "inoculate" the young person against the impact of these messages. The public statements or pledges of intent to abstain are based on research that indicates that sharing intentions with others provides greater compliance.

Evaluations of programs based on the Social Influences Model have been encouraging. Several (Hansen, Malotte, & Fielding, 1988; Johnson, Hansen, Collins, & Graham, 1985; Johnson et al. 1985) have demonstrated reductions in use of cigarettes, alcohol, and marijuana. Research shows that the impact on alcohol use is the most short-lived. This model is designed to respond to ever-changing social influences. Thus, it seems reasonable that the substances impacted, the duration of change, and the ages at which it works may change from time to time as social norms change.

Several additional findings have come from research on this model. One of these findings examined the widely held assumption that multiple years of education are better than just one year. One cohort received Project Smart® in the 6th grade only, with another receiving the intervention annually in the 6th, 7th, and 8th grades. Data were collected three years after the initial implementation (9th grade). Contrary to the prediction, the impact of the curriculum was not greater in the group that received the full program three times. The single administration group had a slight edge with less alcohol and marijuana use. The multiple administration group had a slight edge with less tobacco use (Johnson et al., 1985). However, there were no statistically significant differences. Other research indicates that booster sessions enhance curriculum impact. Together these findings imply that short, follow-up "booster" sessions are helpful, but repetition of the full curriculum every year may not be effective.

Another Project Smart® study (Hansen, Johnson, Flay, Graham, & Sobel, 1988) compared the 12-lesson social influences program with a 12-lesson affective education program. There was a reduction in use by those receiving the social influences program, but an increase in use among those receiving the affective education program. This seems consistent with other research on both approaches.

Research also demonstrated that the approach does not work equally well with all groups and teachers. It seems clear that the model is effective only if implementation follows the necessary criteria of substantial practice by the students and, to a lesser extent, involvement of peer leaders. Project Smart⁸ has shown notable success with these approaches. Project Alert⁸ and Project STAR⁸ were both based on Project Smart⁸ and have also shown positive changes in drug use, though the impact of Project Alert⁸ is short-lived. Project STAR⁸ significantly increased the impact of the approach by incorporating community organization strategies (Pentz et al., 1989).

Not all applications of the model have been effective. Project DARE⁸, which was also derived from Project Smart⁸ and has been widely implemented nationwide, has not shown the same positive results, with the exception of minimal impact on high sensation–seeking youth (Clayton, Cattarello, Day, & Walden, 1991). Project DARE⁸ did not include as many practice sessions as the social influences programs that had greater impact. It also may not include adequate correction of perceptions of the norm, and may include too much affective material. Evaluation of a program called WHOA⁸ indicated that students had more difficulty implementing refusal after the program than before participation in the program (Sehwan, McLeod, & Shantzis, 1989).

PERSONAL AND SOCIAL SKILLS MODEL

The Personal and Social Skills Model, as articulated by Botvin (1990), is an evolutionary step from the two preceding models. Botvin conceptualizes substance abuse, ". . . as a socially learned and functional behavior, resulting from the interplay of social and personal factors . . . learned through modeling and reinforcement, which is influenced by personal factors such as cognitions, attitudes, and beliefs" (p. 495). Programs based on this model incorporate all of the features of the Social Influences Model. These include peer resistance training, teaching awareness of media influences, and activities to change perceptions of the norm. Also, the similarities in goals between this model and affective approaches are striking. The concept of self-esteem illustrates the difference in the two approaches. While affective education emphasizes feelings and achieving increased self-esteem through compliments and building a sense that everyone is special, the Personal and Social Skills Model emphasizes skills and enhancing self-esteem through mastery of the skills. Skill development activities accompany each of the targeted personal and social domains. When practical, the skills are specifically applied to alcohol, drug, and tobacco use, though sometimes they remain generic.

According to Botvin, approaches using this model usually include two or more of the following key elements. The first is general problem-solving and decision-making skills using brainstorming and systematic decision-making techniques. The second is cognitive skills for resisting interpersonal or media influences by identifying the message and developing counterarguments. The third is skills for increasing self-control and self-esteem such as self-instruction, self-reinforcement, goal setting, and self-change. The fourth is adaptive coping strategies for relieving stress or anxiety with cognitive coping skills or behavioral relaxation techniques. The fifth is interpersonal skills such as initiating social interactions, complimenting, or conversation skills; and the sixth is assertiveness skills such as making requests, saying "no," and expressing feelings and opinions. Teaching techniques include instruction, demonstration, feedback, reinforcement, behavior rehearsal during class, and extended practice through behavioral homework assignments. It is best to use follow-up reinforcement sessions. Adults, rather than peer leaders, usually teach these classes.

Botvin, Schenck, and others (Botvin, 1990) have reported outcomes indicating that this approach is superior to the use of the Social Influences Model alone. Evaluations indicate reductions in use of alcohol, tobacco, and marijuana, with results that last at least into high school. Of these substances, the smallest impact was on alcohol use, as was true of the Social Influences Model. It appears that the model demonstrates a way to select, modify, and successfully blend previously used strategies, some of which had already demonstrated effectiveness and some of which had not. However, applications of the model have not been universally successful. One study found that it may be ineffective, or even counterproductive, with abstaining, high-risk teens (Palinkas, Atkins, Miller, & Ferreira, 1996).

We are aware of only one study (Brochu & Souliere, 1988) that applied and measured Botvin's approach to adults. The results were disappointing, underscoring the reality that strategies developed for one age group may not apply across the lifespan. Such outcomes are predictable, since the psychosocial influences involved in initiating alcohol or drug use at one age are not necessarily the same factors involved at another age. This does not diminish the effectiveness of the model; it simply delineates the ages and purposes for which it is useful.

RISK AND RESILIENCY— SOCIAL DEVELOPMENT MODEL

The concept of risk and resiliency has made a major impact on alcohol and drug prevention, and has been widely adopted as the guiding prevention philosophy for many state and federal agencies. The model, as developed by Hawkins and Catalano (Hawkins & Catalano, 1992; Hawkins et al., 1985), takes an approach similar to heart disease prevention in its use of risk reduction factors. This generic model was initially developed as a way to understand and prevent juvenile delinquency and focused only on risk factors. Later, it was expanded to include drug use with added emphasis on the need for communities to work broadly at simultaneously reducing risk factors while increasing protective factors.

Risk Factors

The model identifies five environmental risk factors and 11 individual risk factors that increase the likelihood that an adolescent will use drugs, engage in violent or aggressive behavior, break other laws, or act out sexually.

- Environmental risk factors
  - Economic and social deprivation
  - Low neighborhood attachment and community disorganization
  - Transitions and mobility
  - Community laws and norms favorable toward use
  - Availability
- Individual risk factors
  - Family history of alcoholism
  - Poor family management practices
  - Early antisocial behavior with aggressiveness
  - Parental drug use and positive attitudes toward use
  - Academic failure
  - Low commitment to school
  - Alienation or rebelliousness
  - Antisocial behavior in early adolescence
  - Association with drug-using peers
  - Favorable attitudes toward drugs
  - Early first use of drugs[2]

According to this approach, presence of any of the above risk factors increases likelihood of drug use. Conversely, if risk factors are reduced or removed, use becomes less likely.

Resiliency—Protective Factors

The concept of risk comes from research on common factors among people who developed problems. The concept of resiliency comes from research on common factors among people who avoided major problems, in spite of being raised in an environment that was conducive to developing problems. Protective factors help to de-

---

[2]We refer the reader to Chapter 2. While the association between age of first use and later problems is clearly presented in the literature, other data and the same logic could be used to support the statement that older age of first use is a risk factor for alcoholism. We are not suggesting causality. Instead we are suggesting there is reason to believe that separate bio-psychosocial factors may influence both age of first use and later problems. Thus, age of first use may be more associated with problems without causing the problems.

crease or dampen drug abuse and other problems, even in the face of such negative influences as poverty, chaotic family life, family alcohol or drug problems, or mental illness in parents.

Hawkins and Catalano's Social Development Model (Hawkins et al., 1992) emphasizes bonding as a key protective factor. According to this approach, there are three components to bonding: (1) attachment—positive relationships with others; (2) commitment—an investment in the future; and (3) belief about what is right and wrong. Bonding occurs when three conditions are present. The first is an opportunity to be an active contributor or member of the group. The second is having the skills needed to successfully contribute to the group. The third is a system of consistent recognition as being a contributing, praiseworthy member of the group. Young people who bond strongly to family, peers, and non–drug using peers are less likely to use drugs.

A logical outgrowth of strong bonding is that the person wants to conform to the norms and expectations of that group. Therefore, clear standards for behavior are another important protective factor once bonding is in place. The Social Development Model suggests, then, that we have the strongest chance of preventing adolescent drug use by simultaneously working to remove risk factors and promote bonding with clear expectations.

Bernard (1994) suggests that it is more productive to invest our energies only in protective factors. A focus on resiliency, she suggests, builds what people need to avoid problems regardless of the negative influences that may be present in their lives. She and others have expanded the list of protective factors to include sense of personal control, being loved, sense of meaning, optimism, hope, hardiness, persistence, and a sense of humor. They emphasize the roles of thoughts, attitudes, beliefs, and behaviors in forming the mind and, in some cases, altering biology. They stress that three of the most important tasks of resiliency are finding our way to God, healing our wounds, and expressing our gifts.

Strengths of the Risk and Resiliency Approach

One of the greatest strengths of the risk and resiliency approach is that it has tremendous intuitive appeal. It is also based on a fairly consistent body of research. Also, the model provides an approach to prevention that people can easily understand, and it lends itself well to community activities. Communities using the model can usually select something specific to quickly implement and, as previously noted, this approach has become almost universally adopted by federal, state, and local prevention agencies.

Controlled studies, such as those available for the Social Influences Model or the Personal and Social Skills Model, are not yet available for the risk and resiliency approach. Hawkins' longitudinal study on implementation of parent and teacher training in Seattle schools indicated impact on changing risk factors. However, impact on alcohol or drug use was either nonexistent (Hawkins & Catalano, 1987) or minimal (Hawkins et al., 1989), depending on the group and follow-up point.

Issues about the Risk and Resiliency Approach

Many government and community prevention agencies have adopted the Social Development Model. Therefore, we feel it may be useful to examine more closely some of the issues concerning the model and the concept of risk factors. Figure 4.1 is a graphic

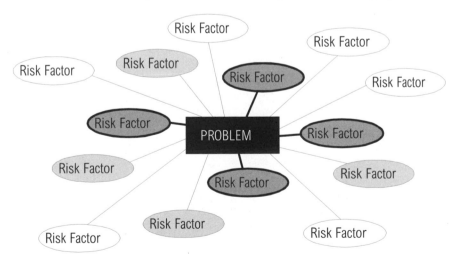

Figure 4.1.   There are many risk factors; changing one or two may not be enough. Also, not all risk factors have equal importance.

representation of the risk portion of the model. As illustrated, a variety of risk factors can impact a person and encourage alcohol or drug abuse. Some risk factors are environmental, while others are internal to the individual. The model suggests that we can prevent abuse by reducing or eliminating the number of risk factors. Resiliency factors could be added to the illustration as shields that protect the person from the risk factors.

Changing Risk Means Changing Risk Factors

In our experience, there are several ways the risk and resiliency approach is being implemented that may not be effective. One approach comes from the penchant of prevention for simply giving information with the hope that knowing translates into doing. We have observed a number of prevention practitioners who believe they are implementing this model when, in fact, they are only going out and teaching about the model. We see no reason to believe that simply teaching the community about the risk and protective factors will do anything to prevent drug use or problems. In order to implement the model, prevention practitioners must bring about change in individual risk and protective factors within individuals and communities—not just talk about the need for change. Successfully applying the model requires broad community organization strategies to reduce risk and develop resiliency.

Changing Only One or Two Factors
May Not Reduce the Problem

Another barrier to implementing this model successfully is that advocates tell communities that reducing *any* risk factor is likely to reduce use. However, there are 16 risk factors in the model and, according to the theory, any one, or any combination, of these risk factors can promote use. It seems logical, then, that one or two risk factors could be completely "eliminated" without making an impact on use due to the presence of other risk factors. As was discussed in Chapter 2, psychosocial influences are like the multiheaded Hydra. Our opinion is that communities must target multiple risk factors, prioritizing them for relative importance.

The Greatest Impact Comes from
the Most Proximal Risk Factors

An additional consideration is that some risk factors are more proximal than others to the actual cause. Most "generic" approaches to prevention are based on the assumption that more distant factors—those not specific to alcohol and drug use—are the "best" focus for prevention. Advocates of generic prevention often cite Jessor and Jessor's Problem Behavior Theory (National Institute on Alcohol Abuse and Alcoholism, 1977) to support their efforts. This work demonstrated that adolescent alcohol and drug abuse does not develop in a vacuum. It often coincides with other initial behaviors including sex, truancy, and engaging in a variety of illegal acts. Their often quoted, and logical, assumption is that the same set of causes or risk factors lead to several different problem behaviors. These risk factors are generic and not specific to any one problem. It also suggests that prevention focused on alcohol- or drug-specific variables such as attitudes about use will not be as effective as activities that are broader in focus. However, the data from which they drew that conclusion demonstrated that the alcohol- and drug-specific variables were more important than the more "generic" factors they suggest targeting.

The Social Development Model assumes that generic changes in poverty, community disorganization, or family management would be as productive as targeting alcohol and drug attitudes. We suggest that positive attitudes about drug use and drug-using peers are more closely related to drug use than is poverty, community disorganization, or family management. For example, people who live in a poorly managed, poverty-ridden home, but who strongly disapprove of drug use, are less likely to use drugs than affluent individuals from well-managed families with favorable attitudes toward use. This is consistent with Bernard's (1994) point that strengthening resiliency—in this case attitudes—is more productive than working on removing risk factors.

Thus, it seems that not all risk factors have equal ability to impact use. Changing those with the most direct impact on use seems more likely to produce results than changing those that less directly affect use. Evaluations of prevention programs seem generally to

support this point. A number of generic, affective education programs improved bonding, raised self-esteem, or improved decision-
making skills, without making any measurable difference on drug
use. On the other hand, peer resistance training specifically targeting
nonuse, and activities that correct misperceptions of norms regarding use, have changed. This is not to say that all generic approaches
are not successful. There are notable exceptions, such as the Perry
School Project (Berrueta-Clement, Schweinhart, Barness, & Weikart, 1983), that demonstrated significant reductions in use. It would
be instructive to analyze the differences in generic programs that
"work" and those that do not. Bernard (1994) suggests that one key
difference is that those generic programs that work tend to focus
more on increasing resiliency than reducing risk. We suggest that,
for both generic and alcohol- and drug-specific prevention, those
that "work best" will target factors that are most proximal to alcohol
and drug use.

People Must Be Able to Do Something about the Risk Factor

Another concern that we have is that, in order to be effective,
prevention strategies must be put into action. When people learn
recommendations for prevention, they need to be able to act on
these. Some risk and resiliency factors are very action-oriented.
Parents and teachers can learn how to promote bonding. Carefully
developed educational campaigns can change favorable attitudes
toward use. Tutoring programs can reduce failure, and new laws can
discourage use. However, some risk factors are difficult, if not
impossible, to act on. For example, how does a community change
its economic situation? How do people change their biological
family histories of alcoholism?

Knowledge about Risk Factors Must Inform Other Actions

Descriptions of this model seem to miss the point that some
risk factors cannot be changed, but can be used to identify groups
that need to be targeted for more intensive prevention. For example,

while we cannot change family history, we can use it to identify people who have increased biological risk. Prevention programs can target these families for more intensive prevention. Knowledge of their biological risk could help them to understand the importance of their drinking choices. Also, we may not be able to prevent children from exhibiting early antisocial behavior, but we can target them for special prevention activities. We do not have the resources necessary to eradicate poverty. It certainly seems beyond the scope of alcohol and drug prevention to do so. However, we can develop targeted prevention programs for those who live in poverty.

Some "Risk Factors" Are Just Correlations

When experts identify something as a risk factor, people assume that it plays a role in causing the problem. The model verifies that interpretation when it suggests that reducing risk factors can reduce the problem. Yet, Hawkins, Lishner, and Catalano (1985) developed the list of risk factors by reviewing correlates of adolescent drug use. The correlates that seemed appropriate to the model's developers were included on the list. By necessity, this was a subjective process. For example, research indicates that, as a group, teens who totally abstain from alcohol and marijuana may be less adjusted socially as young adults then those who minimally use these substances (Newcomb & Butler, 1988), yet no one has suggested good social adjustment is a risk factor, or that poor social adjustment is a protective factor. It is difficult to imagine that this finding would lead to a prevention program designed to make people less socially adjusted. Instead, there are other ways to explain this somewhat troubling finding. Even correlates that are not troubling may not get much attention as risk or protective factors. For example, research clearly indicates that strong religious convictions and active religious participation are strong predictors of abstinence from illegal drugs. In spite of being a stronger predictor than several of the individually listed factors, religious commitment is nearly hidden in general discussions of "bonding to society." Prevention programs do not generally attempt to increase religious commitment. This is predictable, given the important role of government funding in prevention and the controversial nature of church and state issues. All of the correlates that are considered risk factors seem to meet at least two criteria: First, they are consistent with prevailing theories of use; and second, changing them is socially desirable and not controversial. Yet, these two criteria do not assure that the correlates do, in fact, create risk.

Some factors correlate with a condition because they contribute to the cause. For example, being in a tropical area would correlate with development of malaria because it contributes to the cause. Family history of alcoholism and favorable attitudes toward use would appear to be correlates that contribute to the cause of alcoholism.

Other factors correlate with a condition because they have the same "cause" and mutually coexist, but one does not cause the other. This would be like water evaporation and plant growth both occurring faster in sunlight. Evaporation does not cause the plant to grow. Instead, the sun causes both to occur (see Figure 4.2). Children of alcoholics can provide a likely source of this kind of confusion in alcohol and drug research. As discussed, children of alcoholics are about four times more likely to develop alcoholism, even if they are not living with the alcoholic parent. Because of this, anything that is common among children of alcoholics is likely to correlate with alcoholism. Such correlates may or may not play some role in causation. Only research that controls for family history can begin to tell us. For example, childhood sexual abuse is common among women who have alcoholism. It is easy to see how this might contribute to high-risk drinking and thus to alcoholism. On the other hand, a high percentage of daughters of alcoholics are victims of incest. Thus, it is possible that some or all of the increased rate of incest among women with alcoholism could be an effect of being raised with an alcoholic parent. It is possible that being a child of an alcoholic could be a causal factor for both the increased rate of

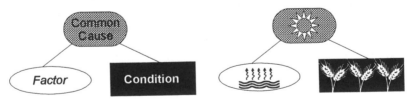

Figure 4.2.   Some risk factors are correlates with a common cause.

incest and the increased rate of alcoholism. In that case, incest would be "baggage" that comes with being a child of an alcoholic, rather than a cause of alcoholism. One study indicated that this is the case (Sher, Gershuny, Peterson, & Raskin, 1997). Additional studies are needed that control for family history. Similar issues could include childhood conduct disorder (which we address below), child abuse, hyperactivity, and learning disabilities.

Research also indicates that children of alcoholics are more likely than children of nonalcoholics to experience drinking-related problems, even when drinking similar amounts. Certain genetic factors may contribute to these problems without causing the alcoholism. For example, there is substantial evidence (Hill & Steinhauer, 1993) that people with increased biological risk for alcoholism may have a low P3 brain wave. People with a lower P3 brain wave have greater difficulty attending to changes in their environment, such as changes in a traffic light (Krein, Overton, Young, Spreier, & Yolton, 1987). There is not yet any indication that the low P3 contributes to risk for alcoholism, although it could contribute to specific alcohol-related problems such as traffic arrests (Begleiter & Kissin, 1996). People who are slow to recognize a changing traffic light, or other changes in the environment, may be especially vulnerable to problems when drinking and driving. It is also possible that the hyperactivity, learning disabilities, and various neurological complications that are more common among children of alcoholics could contribute to this higher incidence of problems.

Correlations also occur when one factor causes another, but our biases may influence our interpretation of which is the cause and which is the effect. For example, depression and alcoholism correlate, and people generally assume the depression causes alcoholism. Research (Schuckit et al., 1990) indicates, though, that while either can develop first, depression more commonly follows alcoholism.

Effective prevention requires these issues to be "sorted out" before assuming that a correlate is a risk factor, and that changing the correlate will reduce risk. For example, since soldiers typically wear green uniforms, it could no doubt be demonstrated that people who wear green during war are more likely to be killed or injured. Yet, all the civilians in the world could avoid wearing green, and the death rate would not be reduced. How might these principles apply to the list of risk factors?

Earlier we raised the possibility that, instead of causing problems, early first use may be caused by the same factors that cause later problems. Rebelliousness, for example, could contribute both to starting use early and to experiencing later problems. If this is the case, then changing age of first use would not contribute significantly to reducing the problem. However, reducing rebelliousness may positively affect both. On the other hand, biological research raises some other interesting possibilities, and may call on us once again to stretch our minds and our models to understand causality more clearly. Even among alcoholics who do not have personality disorders, those who have an early onset (age 25 or younger) tend to have a low turnover rate of serotonin (Virkkunen & Linnoila, 1997). This means the cycle of production and use of this important brain chemical is moving more slowly. Serotonin abnormalities contribute to a variety of behavioral or emotional problems. This research raises the possibility that early onset of problems may be due, in large measure, to biological factors.

Two of the individual risk factors identified by Hawkins and Catalano (1992) involve early antisocial or aggressive behavior, which correlates with early onset of use. The assumption that reducing risk factors reduces risk implies that this early aggressive behavior "causes" later alcohol or drug use. A variety of studies clearly demonstrate that there is a higher proportion of alcohol and drug abuse among those who exhibit early antisocial or aggressive behavior. At first glance, adoption research also seems to provide support for the idea that aggression and antisocial behavior are risk factors. As noted earlier, Cadoret and Gath (1978) identified two factors predictive of alcoholism as adults: a biological parent with alcoholism, or a conduct disorder as a teen. Cloninger et al. (1981) identified two types of alcoholism, one of which was accompanied by early antisocial behavior and aggression; yet, in Cadoret and Gath's adoption study, there was 100 percent overlap between those who had a biological parent with alcoholism and those who had a conduct disorder. Cloninger's Type 2 alcoholism is characterized by early onset and antisocial behavior and appears to be an overlap of alcoholism and antisocial personality disorder. Both have been linked (Virkkunen & Linnoila, 1997) to low serotonin turnover rates. Is early antisocial behavior a risk factor, or does it simply share its biological roots with alcoholism or drug dependence? In either case, will reductions in early aggression prevent later drug abuse? The answers are not clear, but there is reason to believe that early onset of dependence and antisocial behavior mutually coexist, and that preventing aggression may not prevent use.

Another risk factor that has a great deal of intuitive appeal, and a substantial body of supporting research, is family management practices. Again, it is logical to assume that family management practices directly cause teen drug abuse, and that changing family management practices will change teen use. A recent adoption study (McGue, Sharma, & Benson, 1996), which examined teen drinking, had two surprising findings. The first finding showed that the relationship between parental drinking and teen drinking was small and insignificant among adopted offspring, but moderate and significant among birth offspring raised in the same home. This could mean that the inherited biological response to alcohol is a stronger influence on teen drinking than the social influence of parental drinking. Perhaps more surprising was the finding that the relationship between family functioning and teen drinking was modest for the adopted teens, but substantial for birth offspring. This implies that family management practices may not directly influence teen alcohol and drug use. Instead, it is possible that the genetic factors that increase risk for alcoholism or drinking behavior may also affect family management practices, or the two correlates may simply coexist without influencing each other. This second possibility seems consistent with Hawkins' (Hawkins & Catalano, 1987) research, which demonstrates that *Preparing for the Drug-Free Years*, a curriculum based on the risk and resiliency model, did succeed in changing the risk factor of certain family management practices, yet showed no evidence of changing the child's alcohol or drug use.

These unexpected adoption findings are not the only findings which imply that our assumptions may be too simple. For example, children of alcoholics often have difficulty with relationships and have a high rate of divorce. It has been assumed that this is an effect of being raised in a dysfunctional alcoholic home; yet, one study (Goodwin, Schulsinger, Hermansen, Guze, & Winokur, 1973) reported an interesting finding when comparing adoptees who had a biological parent with alcoholism and those who did not. The biological children of alcoholics, raised with nonalcoholic adoptive parents, had unusually high divorce rates compared to other adoptees. This was even true when they did not develop alcoholism. While these findings may seem implausible, it is important to keep in mind that many personality traits appear to be 40 percent to 60 percent heritable (Cloninger, Sigvardsson, & Bohman, 1988). Many of us notice that our children have personality traits, preferences, or mannerisms similar to grandparents or other relatives with whom they have spent little time; most of us have little difficulty attributing this to heredity. However, that awareness has been slow to find its way into theories of behavior. Some of the psychosocial "risk factors" may not contribute to causality, even if they fit nicely into prevailing theory and assumptions.

Identified Risk Factors Are Not Universal

Except for the adoption research, the studies used to support the Hawkins and Catalano model were on young people who used illicit drugs at an early age. In practice, however, the model is often applied as though these risk factors are relevant to all substances and ages. This assumption may not be warranted. For example, if we look at college students in general, and fraternity members in particular, most of the model does not apply. Fraternity members often have significant financial resources. They are often highly attached and bonded to their fraternities, campuses, and families. Most are succeeding academically, and all are surrounded by laws and school policies governing use of alcohol. They often come from well-managed families, did not present early antisocial behavior or aggressiveness, have a high commitment to school, and are not alienated. Yet it is not unusual to find 70 percent or more reporting (Thompson, 1996) that they have had 13 or more drinks on one or more days in the past month. Only two of the risk factors routinely apply: They have attitudes that favor alcohol use and peers that use. However, the model generally does not apply, and the group members see themselves as more protected than at increased risk.

If our prevention intentions extend beyond childhood users and illicit drugs, then it seems important to recognize that large numbers of adult alcohol, tobacco, and prescription drug abusers only minimally fit the risk factor approach. This is not intended as a criticism of the model, only as a recognition of its limitations. It is important not to extend a model beyond what it was developed to represent and accomplish. The research supporting the model was drawn from populations of early, illicit drug users. It seems most reasonable, then, to assume that these are risk factors for early illicit drug use, and maintain the likely possibility that the model does not necessarily apply to all substances and all ages.

Risks We Can Change and Risks We Cannot Change

Finally, Hawkins and Catalano (1992) suggest that their Social Development Model (Risk and Resiliency) mirrors heart disease prevention since both focus on reducing risk factors. They suggest that the overall success of heart disease prevention, and of specific projects such as the Stanford Three Communities Study (Maccoby et al., 1977), are indications that the Social Development Model can be effective for alcohol and drug problems. We suggest there is a major difference between the Social Development Model risk factors approach and the risk factors approach used for heart disease. As noted in the previous chapter, heart disease risk factors are divided into risks we cannot change—which are biological—and risks we can change—which are behavioral. All the risk factors targeted by heart disease prevention are *behavioral* risk factors—those within the control of the individual. Heart disease prevention theory recognizes that psychological and social factors play a role in etiology and prevention, but they are not "treated" as risk factors.

In contrast, of the 16 risk factors targeted by the Social Development model, only "family history of alcoholism" is listed as partially biological. The only behavior the targeted individual can change is early initial use. The other factors are psychosocial factors, which cannot be acted on, or changed, by the individual. Heart disease prevention targets individuals to change. The Social Development Model targets the community to change. Even in community trials, such as the Stanford Three Communities Study, the focus of community-wide action was to support individual behavior change, not to change community economic levels or cohesiveness. In the Lifestyle Risk Reduction Formula, the focus of heart disease prevention is awareness of biological risk and individual behavior change in the behavioral, quantity/frequency risk. In the Social Development Model, the emphasis is on the psychosocial influences. The Social Development approach is somewhat like heart disease prevention in that both target risk factors. However, the Social Development theory approaches the entire concept of risk and risk factors differently.

The Social Development Model makes important contributions to prevention thinking. However, if the focus is only on "risk factors" that are actually psychosocial influences, then we are missing much of the potential impact of prevention. For example, family disorganization does not directly cause alcohol or drug addiction, but quantity and frequency of use, in combination with an individual's biology, does contribute.

The Lifestyle Risk Reduction formula (see Fig. 3.2) and Schuckit and Smith's research (1996) described earlier (see Chapter 3) provide good examples of this. Sixty percent of college-age people who had both a family history of alcoholism and a high tolerance qualified for a DSM-III diagnosis of either alcohol abuse or alcohol dependence within nine years. Family history of alcoholism and high tolerance to the impairment effects of alcohol are two indicators of increased biological risk, represented in the biology part of the Lifestyle Risk Reduction formula. We are not aware of any of the psychosocial risk factors that have this predictive power.

The importance of heredity in the development of alcoholism has been well documented since the 1970s. It is time to integrate heredity clearly as a powerful risk factor with straightforward guidance about preventive actions to be taken. We need to broaden the concept of risk from psychosocial risk factors to bio-psychosocial risk. Although all three factors influence one another, there is one, even more important, universal risk factor. In order to understand it, we need to shift our concept of the purpose of prevention from being the prevention of use to being the prevention of problems. Once we make that shift, it becomes clear that high-risk use is the greatest, and most universal, risk factor. Of all the risk factors, it is the one that is most under each individual's control.

Looking again at Schuckit and Smith's research (1996) and other longitudinal studies, it is easy to see that only those who were making high-risk drinking choices developed alcohol-related problems. Those who were abstaining, or making other low-risk choices during the study, did not develop alcohol problems, even if they had high tolerance and a positive family history. Choices are represented in the quantity/frequency behavior portion of the Lifestyle Risk Reduction formula. Drinking or drug-taking behavior is not included in most models of etiology and, thus, omitted from prevention. In a general sense, it is easy to believe that psychosocial, or even bio-psychosocial factors, cause "alcohol and drug problems." In a specific sense, it is not possible to seriously maintain that they alone cause physical addiction, cirrhosis, impairment-related crashes, or any other specific problem. Quantity/frequency choices are part of the etiology of any specific use-related problem.

As previously mentioned, the Social Development Model has been adopted by many federal, state, and local prevention agencies as their central prevention philosophy. It is a model that has much to offer. However, using it, or any of the other youth-focused models as the central guiding philosophy will ignore several important factors. For example, if a community implemented the model exactly as designed, that community may take action on any of a variety of "risk factors" to reduce childhood drug use. These issues may include family management, bonding, family and community cohesiveness, or eradication of poverty. At the same time, however, people who do not live in poverty, do not have a family history of alcoholism, do not support illegal drug use, and do have a relatively well-managed family will feel quite secure. Even those who have a family history of alcoholism are likely to feel confident, as long as they have avoided family chaos. In addition, adults will learn the importance of abstinence for kids, but they will not be made aware of the need to reduce high-risk alcohol and drug behaviors across the lifespan. Neither will they learn how to estimate biological risk for themselves or their children, or the quantities of drinking that will present risk in their own lives. For example, adults who drink a half-dozen drinks throughout an evening will not be given any reason to be concerned for their own health. The model simply does not address these important issues. Instead, the approach will focus the community on only one part of the lifespan—on illegal drugs or underage drinking—and on one part of the formula—on psychosocial factors. Community members will no doubt be surprised if an alcohol- or drug-related problem develops and will wonder how it could have happened since they did not fit "the profile." Lifetime prevention is much more than controlling the psychosocial risk factors for adolescent use of illicit drugs.

There is no doubt that a variety of psychosocial risk factors are compelling influences on adopting high-risk behaviors. Each person has the power to rise above these influences and choose a low-risk lifestyle. There is no doubt that prevention should embrace psychosocial influences. However, it seems equally important to keep people focused on the single risk factor that has the most direct and controlling role in either triggering or preventing problems: quantity and frequency behavior. Anyone who wants to reduce risk for alcohol- or drug-related problems for a lifetime can do so regardless of any of their biological or psychosocial risk factors; doing so requires understanding the nature of risk and the role of behavior in creating risk.

5

Behavior

The Ultimate Risk and Protective Factor

Everyone is trying to accomplish something big, not realizing that life is made up of little things.
—Frank A. Clark

Alcohol- and drug-related problems are complex, and most models focus on parts of etiology and prevention. Some of these models are very specific, targeting one age cohort or one aspect of etiology, while others are broader. We believe there are advantages to using a model that is broad enough to integrate several, more narrowly focused models. To us, both the Public Health Model and the Lifestyle Risk Reduction Model are broad enough to encompass other models. In particular, the Lifestyle Risk Reduction Model has the precision to show how the more targeted, youth-focused models fit into the bigger picture.

THINKING BROADLY: THE PUBLIC HEALTH TRIANGLE

The Public Health Model, a non–problem-specific model, is generic to all health problems and has been broadly applied to alcohol and drug problems for over 20 years. The model proposes three components to any health problem: the *agent*—exemplified by the bacteria, virus, chemical, or any other triggering agent for a health problem; the *host*—the human that develops the health problem; and the *environment*—the setting which brings the agent and host together. Since all three components are necessary for a problem to occur, action to prevent the problem can be taken at any of the three levels. For example, the host can be removed from exposure or "strengthened" by inoculation or fluoridation. The agent can be removed by killing mosquitoes that spread infection, killing bacteria, removing sources of radiation, or removing alcohol or drugs. The environment can be altered so that the agent and host are not "brought together" by, for example, draining swamps that breed mosquitoes, cleaning up water supplies that harbor bacteria, or changing laws to make alcohol or drugs less accessible.

The appeal of the Public Health Model is universality. It applies to all health problems and many nonhealth problems, thus providing universal and generic ways of intervening. On the other hand, because it is not problem-specific, it must be linked with a problem-specific model before it can be made useful. Heart disease and malaria both easily fit the Public Health Model, but another model is needed to understand that malaria is caused by a bacteria carried by mosquitoes. Only then do we know what action to take with the agent, host, or environment. Similarly, only when we understand that heart disease is a lifestyle-related health problem, do we understand what action to take to prevent it.

The first and most formative alcohol-specific model that was used with the Public Health Model was the Distribution of Consumption Model. That model proposed that consumption is distributed proportionately at all times, so that changes in per capita consumption would be related to similar percent reductions in light, moderate, and heavy drinkers. Therefore, policy measures to restrict availability of alcohol should reduce all levels of use simultaneously, including heavy use and, subsequently, use-related problems.

It was logical to apply the Public Health Model with the Distribution of Consumption Model, using environmental policy changes such as increased taxes, reduced sales outlets, advertising restrictions, and warning labels for alcohol. For many people, the Public Health Model seems synonymous with these actions. In reality, the Public Health Model is much broader. The Lifestyle

Risk Reduction Model is a way of widely operationalizing the Public Health Model.

INTEGRATING PREVENTION FOR A LIFETIME: FIVE CONDITIONS OF LIFESTYLE RISK REDUCTION

The Five Principles of Lifestyle Risk Reduction (see Chapter 3) are related to five conditions that must be present, or developed, for a successful risk reduction effort (see Table 5.1). The challenge

Table 5.1.   Five Principles and Five Conditions of Lifestyle Risk Reduction

Principle One: Everyone has biological risk.	**Condition One:** People believe that alcohol and drug problems could happen to them and understand that quantity of alcohol and drugs used and frequency of intake are the only factors standing between them and a problem. (It could happen to me; my choices matter.)
Principle Two: The quantity and frequency of specific choices create risk.	**Condition Two:** People learn how to estimate their level of biological risk and learn what specific quantity and frequency behavior are high risk and low risk. (I know what to do.)
Principle Three: The level of biological risk determines the quantity and frequency that will be high risk.	**Condition Three:** An environment has been fostered that supports low-risk choices with norms, expectations, laws, policies, and messages from informal and formal groups such as family, friends, media, workplace, religious groups, school, community, and government. (People around me support low-risk choices.)
Principle Four: Health problems occur when the level of high-risk choices "matches" the level of biological risk.	**Condition Four:** People develop commitment to making low-risk choices and hold attitudes, values, and self-concepts that support adoption of low-risk choices. (I want to make low-risk choices.)
Principle Five: Social and psychological factors influence quantity and frequency choices.	**Condition Five:** People develop skills that will allow them to implement low-risk choices in their daily lives. (I have the skills I need.)

for the prevention practitioner is to establish these conditions at the individual or community level. We will introduce the five conditions specifically worded for alcohol and drugs. However, they apply to all lifestyle-related problems and could be stated generically, or reworded to apply to any specific problem.

Condition One: "It Could Happen to Me; My Choices Matter"

People believe that alcohol and drug problems could happen to them and understand that the quantity of alcohol and drugs used, and frequency of intake, are the only factors standing between them and a problem.

Those in the addiction field talk a great deal about denial. As typically discussed, it refers to an individual's denial of an existing problem through the use of defense mechanisms. These denial mechanisms are a major focus of both intervention and recovery. Yet, there is another form of denial that is experienced by even more people. This prevention denial is experienced by people who do not have the problem and believe that the problem could never happen to them.

Prevention denial is the seed of later denial. Because people believe that they could not develop a problem, it is easy to believe that it has not happened. This denial represents one of the biggest barriers to successful prevention activities. Until people believe that the problem could happen to them, they are not likely to take prevention programs seriously. The logic is simple but flawed: "If the problem cannot happen to me, then I do not need to do anything to prevent it." One of the most common ways we have of supporting and maintaining this denial is through the development of a belief structure that the problem can only happen to certain kinds of people who are "not like me." This keeps prevention impersonal, external, and largely irrelevant to anyone who holds this view.

The first condition of Lifestyle Risk Reduction addresses prevention denial. It personalizes prevention and shifts the locus of control for prevention directly to the person in such a way that the person can take action. Risk for the problem is moved from something "out there" that happens to "people unlike me," to something very internal and personal. There are two forms of risk: those risks each person cannot control—biology—and those a person can control—quantity and frequency of alcohol or drug use. Since none of us can control our biology, we must make low-risk choices to avoid problems. Our psychological makeup and our social environment will make this task easier or harder, but it is up to each of us to make low-risk choices. Even if there are high-risk influences in our environment that we cannot change, we can still choose to make low-risk choices. Prevention is actionable. It is within our control.

Most Americans grow up understanding that heart disease could happen to anyone. They know that some people have increased biological risk and that our choices can either protect us or create greater risk. A heart disease prevention program does not need to spend much time with Condition One. But for alcoholism and drug dependence, the situation is very different. Our culture supports the idea that alcoholism and other alcohol-related problems happen only to certain kinds of people. People widely believe that personal strength, or the ability to "handle it," is more important than how much or how often they drink or use drugs.

Unfortunately, prevention efforts can unwittingly play into those beliefs, deepening the denial. One way this happens is by overemphasizing high-risk *groups* to the public. For example, affective education has been successful in convincing many people that low self-esteem is the *cause* of problems. As a result, people with high self-esteem often see no need for adopting preventive *behaviors*. Another example comes from early AIDS education which emphasized that the high-risk *groups* were homosexual males and intravenous drug users. The result was that people outside these groups felt they did not have to worry about AIDS. Only later did AIDS prevention focus on high-risk *behaviors* independent of group affiliation. An even more dangerous variation on this theme, used throughout the health field, is the reference to "at-risk groups." If one group is "at risk," then what is everyone else? The apparent answer is "not at risk." "If I am not at risk, I do not need to worry about prevention." We fear that alcohol and drug prevention is in danger of repeating these mistakes. There is a growing emphasis on high-risk groups and increasing discussion of being "at risk" in alcohol and drug prevention programs.

Our earlier discussion of college fraternities provides a good example of a group that believes they have little risk. A survey conducted by one national fraternity revealed that the vast majority of its national membership indicated that alcohol was a *problem on campus,* both for those who belonged to fraternities, and those who did not. However, even though they reported heavy drinking and multiple alcohol-related problem incidents in their chapters, the members still did not see alcohol as a *problem in their chapter.* The problem was "out there." In subsequent interactions with these groups, they repeatedly referred to their high self-esteem, good grades, high caliber of members, and long lists of accomplishments as proof that they did not have to worry about their drinking. This was stated despite the fact that members were getting arrested for drinking, having injuries related to drinking, and being put on probation by school officials for alcohol-related incidences. They seemed to be saying, "Yes we drink a lot, and problem incidences have occurred, but these are nothing that we can't handle. We know we don't have to worry because we are the kind of people who do not develop problems with alcohol. We are protected by our strengths." Students supported these beliefs by remembering what they had been taught in junior high or high school prevention programs about self-esteem, good grades, commitment to school, and bonding with "mainstream organizations." According to these criteria, they were "not at risk," so their own behavior did not seem to be a particular problem. Their concern was avoiding immediate problem incidences, so they focused on designated drivers and other preventive activities that did not interfere with their drinking. The prevention programs they had encountered earlier did not deal with drinking, but with abstinence and psychosocial factors. Unfortunately, this prevention convinced them they were safe, and that their quantity and frequency choices did not matter.

Establishing Condition One—helping people believe that alcohol and drug problems could happen to them—can take time, even under the best of circumstances. It takes even longer if it is necessary to overcome the effects of previous prevention messages. The more deeply entrenched a person is in making high-risk choices, the more time it may take to establish Condition One. Until Condition One is in place, though, there is little reason to proceed with prevention.

Any viewpoint that attributes the cause of the problem to any single factor, or to any combination of factors that does not include use, may convince people that their choices are of little consequence. These beliefs must be convincingly and persuasively challenged before people can seriously consider a new way of thinking. Once this is accomplished, we find an understanding of the Lifestyle Risk Reduction formula to be useful in completing this condition (see Fig. 3.2). Successfully establishing Condition One requires skill in selecting content and mastery of the art of persuasion, both of which are discussed in Chapter 6.

In theory, any alcohol- or drug-related problem could be used to establish Condition One in an educational program. People incorrectly assume that with youth, prevention must focus on immediate problem outcomes. For alcohol, then, we are often told to focus on drunk driving, date rape, or school failure. The belief is that young people are not concerned about long-term health problems such as addiction or physical damage. Yet, according to the *Monitoring the Future* Surveys (Johnston et al., 1996), and to the National Survey of American Attitudes on Substance Abuse (Kaftarian, Kingery, & Mains, 1997), fear of physical damage or addiction are the primary reasons young people give for not using drugs. This fits with our experience, which we will address under Condition Four. Focusing on health problems as the means of establishing Condition One has the benefit of being of concern to most people, as well as having the richest body of research from which it can be established that there are risks beyond the control of the person making high-risk choices. It may be more difficult to establish a sense of vulnerability to high-risk choices when using fights, date rape, or other interpersonal problems as the initial focus. Data on how frequent these problems are, and how closely tied they are to high-risk choices, are not likely to make an impact on perception of risk as long as the view, "I can handle it," goes unchallenged. With social problems, people can always hold on to the belief that they can manage their behavior, even when drunk. When biological risk is explained, people can easily understand that this is beyond their control. Once that vulnerability is established, it can then be generalized to other problems.

When people internalize that alcoholism, drug dependence and other use-related problems are personal, and that their quantity/frequency choices are the only thing standing between them and a problem, prevention takes on a new sense of urgency, and they want to know what they can do to prevent these problems. Once people reach this point, they are ready for Condition Two.

Condition Two: "I Know What to Do"

People learn how to estimate their level of biological risk and learn what specific quantity and frequency behaviors are high risk and low risk.

The focus of the first condition is that both biological risk and quantity/frequency choices are important. The second condition states that people need to know specific information to prevent problems. If behavior is the ultimate risk factor, then Condition Two could be considered the ultimate condition. It empowers people with the reality that, "I know what to do." Drug abuse prevention has always incorporated one form of quantity/frequency–specific guidance—zero use. Alcohol abuse prevention has usually incorporated the same advice for those under legal age, but for adults who drink, it has relied on vague guidance such as, "drink moderately," "drink responsibly," or "drink socially." Thus, each person has been able to define these terms however he or she chooses, which has led to problems. Most people can see that this kind of guidance would have been useless for heart disease prevention. Imagine, for example, that heart disease prevention programs had replaced the specific information they provide on exercise and diet with general admonitions to eat "moderate" amounts of dietary fat and exercise "responsibly." The likelihood of that translating into "30 minutes of aerobic exercise three times a week," and "servings of steak the size of a deck of cards" is slim. But somehow people have expected that admonitions to "drink responsibly" would be sufficient to prevent alcohol-related problems. People need more specificity.

Several quantity/frequency guidelines have been proposed over the past several years. Most do not involve any estimation of biological risk and fall short of what is needed to establish Condition Two—"I know what to do." The first effort to teach specific quantity/frequency guidelines may have been blood alcohol charts, graphs, and wheels that are still used today. Many of us first saw these devices in health education textbooks, drivers' manuals, or as wallet cards. These charts allow people to look up their body weight and the number of drinks consumed and see the estimated blood alcohol level that will result. While easy to use, the charts are misleading. They are based on the average rate of alcohol metabolism which is usually considered to be one-half ounce per hour. The true average is somewhat less than that but, more importantly, the range of alcohol metabolism is from one-quarter ounce to one full ounce per hour (Begleiter & Kissin, 1996). Thus, people who are one-quarter ounce metabolizers will be underestimating by as much as 100 percent! Their blood alcohol level will be twice as high as the chart indicates. In addition, the charts use total body weight when the real issue is total body water, again causing underestimation of risk. Finally, the charts do not take into account other factors that can affect either blood alcohol level or impairment, such as stomach content, gender, altitude, medication, tiredness, or illness. The result can be serious miscalculations. It is not unusual for those who work with DUI offenders to hear, "I followed my chart exactly, and I still got arrested." Is this rationalization? Perhaps; but it can also be true. Another problem with blood alcohol charts is that, by using blood alcohol levels as the ultimate measure, focus is taken away from health problems entirely and shifted to impairment problems. When using a chart, a person can conclude that it would be low risk to drink amounts that can create serious risk for health problems over time. Several journal articles (O'Neill, Williams, & Dubowski, 1983) have recommended against using charts. We agree.

A variety of other low-risk guidelines have also been recommended, most of which range from one to three drinks per day. Former surgeon general C. Everett Koop recommended no more than two drinks per day as being low risk, as has the Addiction Research Foundation in Canada. The United States Department of Agriculture issued guidelines of no more than two per day for men and one per day for women. The British guidelines have recently been revised from weekly amounts to daily amounts of two to three drinks per day for women, and three to four per day for men. All of these guidelines have some grounding in research and are straightforward, but none consider *all* the important variables.

Following an extensive review of several hundred studies on alcohol-related morbidity and mortality, Prevention Research Institute saw a need for multilevel guidelines that incorporate different levels of biological risk, differences for daily drinkers or nondaily drinkers, and adjustments for individual differences that affect impairment. These guidelines are incorporated in a five step risk reduction process (Daugherty & O'Bryan, 1986, 1996) that allows each individual to apply all relevant factors, determine their low-risk range, and to consider other factors such as laws, job or school policies, personal and family values, and religious beliefs, to assure a choice that does not lead to social problems. The definition of "a drink" is based on one-half ounce of absolute alcohol which translates into 12 ounces of 4 to 5 percent beer, 4 ounces of 12 percent wine, or 1 ounce of 100 proof spirits.

The guidelines begin by identifying three levels of biological risk. For the lowest level of risk (no family history of alcoholism and no high tolerance), the guidelines identify up to two drinks in any day as being low risk for those who drink on most days, and up to three drinks for those who do not drink daily. Since any drinking that leads to impairment is high risk, even if it is otherwise within the low-risk range, special recommendations are given to adjust for such individual differences as body size, gender, altitude, medication, illness, tiredness, empty stomach, and age. The second level of risk is for those who have *either* high tolerance or one family member with alcoholism. These guidelines are to avoid daily drinking with no more than two drinks in any day. For those with both a family history of alcoholism *and* high tolerance to alcohol, or for those with multiple relatives with alcoholism, the recommended guideline is total abstinence.

The final guideline can be hard for people to accept if they meet the criteria and enjoy drinking. Total abstinence is widely accepted as a recovery guideline for people who already have alcoholism, or as prevention advice for children. But accepting abstinence as a prevention for adults who do not have alcoholism can be a struggle. Schuckit's and Smith's research (1996; reviewed earlier) is just one example of the wisdom of abstinence for those who have both a family history of alcoholism and a high tolerance to alcohol. Since 60 percent of Schuckit's sample developed a diagnosis of alcohol abuse or dependence before age 30, it is difficult to recommend anything other than abstinence for this group.

On the other hand, there are those who believe that anyone who has a parent with alcoholism should abstain. They believe the guideline of zero to two drinks and not daily is too liberal for those who have either high tolerance or one relative with alcoholism, but not both. Adoption research (Goodwin, 1984) indicates that about one-fourth of the biological children of alcoholics developed alcoholism, and Schuckit and Smith (1996) reported 15 percent for those who did not have high tolerance to alcohol. It should be noted that overall population data for a diagnosis of alcohol abuse or dependence among males age 18–30 is not much different. This, combined with the lack of evidence that zero to two drinks and less than daily drinking increase risk for problems, seems to indicate that the guideline is adequately conservative.

Following the low-risk guidelines will reduce all three types of problems—health, impairment, and social. Also, Prevention Research Institute's Five Step Risk Reduction Process puts low-risk guidelines within the context of laws, family and religious values, and expectations. This provides information for a lifetime within the context of age-appropriate expectations. Thus, young people receive life-saving information for their lifetime without undercutting societal or parental expectations for abstinence. Still, experience suggests that the very mention of teaching such information to young people will be anxiety-provoking for some readers, who fear it is not possible to teach about low-risk guidelines without undercutting the goal of abstinence for youth. We believe it is important to understand more about the model before dealing with this issue. For now, we ask the reader to at least temporarily consider that experience indicates this approach will increase rates of abstinence and decrease high-risk use among students in junior high school and high school, college age youth, and adults. We will address the issue in more depth in Chapter 7.

Condition Two—"I know what to do"—may be the ultimate condition, but it must be used in conjunction with Condition One—"It could happen to me"—or it is useless. People can be repeatedly told what constitutes low-risk behaviors, but they are not likely to adopt these behaviors if they believe the problem really results from the kind of person they are rather than the kind of choices they make. In fact, providing guidelines before a person is ready to hear them may work against their ultimate adoption, insuring the information a "so what" or a "been there, done that" response. However, after Condition One is understood and internalized, a person will ask for specific information. At that point, its sense of novelty can assist in the process of changing behavior. Only when Condition One is accepted, are low-risk guidelines useful.

We have found that former surgeon general Koop's admonition to drink no more than two drinks per day is relatively well known, yet we find no evidence that people changed their drinking as a result of their knowledge. The surgeon general's good efforts would represent an attempt to accomplish Condition Two without first accomplishing Condition One. We urge patience. Condition One must preceded Condition Two, not only for individuals but for groups.

Conditions One and Two are the core of the Lifestyle Risk Reduction Model and set it apart from other alcohol and drug prevention models. We are not aware of any other models that incorporate Conditions One and Two and, according to the Lifestyle Risk Reduction approach, effective prevention is unlikely until they are achieved. The first condition sets the stage for the second condition, and each of the remaining three conditions support the second condition. As Table 5.2 illustrates, Conditions Three, Four, and Five are not unique to Lifestyle Risk Reduction, except in relating them to the first two conditions.

Condition Three: "People around Me Support Low-Risk Choices"

An environment has been fostered that supports low-risk choices with norms, expectations, laws, policies, and messages from informal and formal groups such as family, friends, media, workplace, religious groups, school, community, and government.

In a perfect world, the environment would be supportive of low-risk choices and prevention would be easily accomplished. Needless to say, this is not a perfect world. Prevention practitioners face the difficult task of reshaping an environment that often "works against" preventing alcohol and drug problems into one that is more

Table 5.2.   How Youth-Oriented Models Integrate with the Five Conditions of Lifestyle Risk Reduction

Lifestyle Risk Reduction	Social Development	Social Influences	Personal and Social Skills
Condition One: It could happen to me, my choices matter.	Not addressed	Not addressed	Not addressed
Condition Two: I know what to do.	Not addressed	Not addressed	Not addressed
Condition Three: People around me support low-risk choices.	P Clear norms & laws R Economic & social deprivation R Community disorganization R Transitions & mobility R Availability R Alcoholic family R Poor family management	Not addressed	Not addressed
Condition Four: I want to make low-risk choices.	P Bonded to family, church, school, society R Early antisocial R Academic failure R Low commitment R Alienation R Rebelliousness R Antisocial teen R Prouse attitudes R Early first use	Correct misperceptions of norms	Increase self-esteem Increase decision-making ability
Condition Five: I have the skills I need.	Not addressed	Peer resistance Media analysis	Assertiveness skills Anxiety reduction Communication Resisting media & personal influence Social skills

P = Protective factor; R = Risk factor

prevention-friendly. This task is not new. In fact, a large portion of the prevention efforts during the 1980s and 1990s was directed toward this goal. Advocates of the Public Health Model focused their efforts on raising alcohol and tobacco taxes, restricting advertising, raising the legal purchase age, increasing penalties, requiring drug testing, and implementing other policy measures designed to reduce per capita consumption. There have also been major efforts to build public support for a consistent abstinence message for youth.

The difference in the Lifestyle Risk Reduction approach is that Conditions One and Two guide efforts to change the environment. The first environmental change targeted within the Lifestyle Risk Reduction Model approach is establishing a new way of thinking about the cause of alcohol and drug problems. Condition Three—"People around me support low-risk choices"—brings the focus of Condition One—"It could happen to me"—to a level of common thought. There is broad understanding that these problems could happen to anyone, and that making low-risk choices is the only way to protect ourselves from problems. When successful, this "new view" becomes the "prevailing view," replacing "old views." People no longer think they can make high-risk choices with relative impunity as long as they are the right kind of people.

Once Condition One—"It could happen to me"—is common thought, people are ready to learn about low-risk behaviors identified in Condition Two—"I know what to do." Thus, the environmental prevention strategies focused on establishing new norms are broadened to include the lifespan and all three goals: increase abstinence, delay onset of use, and reduce high-risk use.

The Lifestyle Risk Reduction Model proposes that environmental prevention efforts target support of abstinence for youth, as well as establish expectations and support for low-risk behaviors by adults. Instead of adults simply taking a position on what youth should do, adults would begin to examine their own choices more closely and support an environment that encourages low-risk behaviors at all ages, thus giving the message, "In this society (community, family, religious group), we all make age-appropriate low-risk choices that are consistent with our values." For everyone, this includes abstinence from illegal drugs; following the directions for medications; and following age-appropriate low-risk guidelines for alcohol. For those under legal age, abstinence from alcohol will be the only low-risk choice consistent with the law, and for those over legal age, low-risk choices depend on the level of biological risk. For religious groups that only accept abstinence from alcohol, the message is, "Abstinence is the only low-risk choice consistent with our beliefs." For other religious groups, other low-risk choices could be acceptable. The unifying message that transcends the lifespan is that for all substances and all groups "age-appropriate low-risk choices are consistent with our values."

When people think about changing public thinking, the media usually comes to mind as the tool of choice. Certainly, both media and community organization strategies play an important role in Condition Three. However, small group education is also important. Many of the beliefs and attitudes, as well as much of the understanding necessary to accomplish this condition, take time and intense, structured efforts to accomplish.

Condition Four: "I Want to Make Low-Risk Choices"

People develop commitment to making low-risk choices and hold attitudes, values, and self-concept that support adoption of low-risk choices.

For some people, commitment to a low-risk lifestyle happens easily. For others, it is harder. The second group presents a challenge. How do we structure prevention in a way that encourages commitment and the attitudes, values, and self-concept that support it?

In our experience, one step in this process is making the risks real. People often comment that young people feel invulnerable and believe they will live forever. Because of this, many people believe that a risk reduction approach will not work with young people. That does not fit our experience. Young people seem to take more risks than older people; however, they do not take risks indiscriminately. Their behavior seems indiscriminate to adults because they take risks that we would not take. For the most part, when the risk is real to them—when they believe that behavior "A" is likely to lead to undesirable outcome "B"—they are no more likely to take the risk than are most adults. The problem is that risk often is not perceived as real to the young person. They have not had enough "near-miss experiences," or friends who have experienced death or injury, to fully understand the risk. Also, they may respond to peer challenges to do something risky even if they are afraid. In this instance, their fear of being perceived as weak is greater than their fear of the risk. Perhaps this happens more to teens, at least in part, because a teen peer group is more likely to challenge and taunt than is an adult peer group.

After years of lifestyle risk reduction education with young people, we find that their response to the question, "What was most meaningful to you?" is often the same as adults' response. Most will say, "Discovering that alcoholism could happen to me," and "Learning what was low risk for me." These evaluative statements are supported by the *Monitoring the Future* Survey, which indicates that increased perception of risk preceded the national decrease in marijuana use by teens, and decreased perception of risk preceded the more recent increase in use. Our goal, then, is to make these risks real to people of all ages.

A second step in developing commitment to low-risk choices is to help people assess what they value most and understand how high-risk choices endanger those valued objects, while low-risk choices protect them. With the possible exception of the most alienated or antisocial individuals, the vast majority of people value family, health, freedom, and self-respect. But just as the risks of our behavior may not be real to us, the extent to which our behaviors jeopardize our deepest values may not be apparent. Once this becomes clear, we are back to making the risk real: that individual high-risk choices are likely to ultimately take away "my freedom, my health, my finances, or my family." This is taking, "It could happen to me" to a new level. Now it is not just alcoholism or drug dependence that "could happen to me"—it is the loss of "what I value most in life." This is illustrated by a conversation with a college student who had been raised in a single-parent home. When asked why he had never used drugs, he quickly replied, "Oh, it would have broken my mother's heart!" The relationship with his mother was clearly more important to him than any pleasure that would have been derived from drugs. Also important is that she had apparently made that link clear for him. Another example comes from research on "spontaneous remission" in alcohol or drug dependence. Spontaneous remission is the term used to describe those situations where problematic use suddenly stops without apparent therapeutic intervention. The most frequent situations preceding such "spontaneous" events were religious conversion experiences, beginning a new love relationship, or an ultimatum from a loved spouse or significant other: "Either the drinking goes or I go." In each case, it was clear to the person that something else meant more and that their continued use was going to destroy it.

Another closely related aspect of encouraging commitment to making low-risk choices is helping people feel compassion, concern, love, support, high expectations, and respect from people who expect them to make low-risk choices. One experiment with medical students illustrates this power. Each student in the experimental group was assigned a faculty member who wrote a weekly letter to the student giving support, encouragement, and caring. Even though this was the limit of the relationship, it seemed to be enough to make a statistically significant reduction in the drinking by the experimental group compared to controls who did not receive such support.

Also important is an opportunity for people to identify with individuals and groups that expect low-risk choices of them, and to make a meaningful contribution to the lives of these people and groups. This creates bonding. The need for bonding is an important aspect of both affective education and resiliency approaches. The benefit of bonding should be self-evident, but it is important that bonding not be seen as magical, in and of itself. Fraternity members often share deep bonds, but often make very high-risk drinking choices. The previously mentioned research at the Addiction Research Foundation (Shain et al., 1980) indicated that bonding between parent and child could be increased but, contrary to the theory, it did not decrease use. Instead, it increased the chance that the children would adopt the same behavior as their parents, which could increase use. For this reason, Prevention Research Institute took a different approach to parent education in which the program made a concerted effort to bring the parents' drinking within a low-risk range before asking parents to focus on their children. This approach led to a decrease in high-risk drinking by parents and an increase in abstinence and decrease in high-risk drinking in their children (Thompson, 1996). Thus, each of us must be bonded to people and groups that expect low-risk behaviors of us in order for the bonding to promote commitment to low-risk choices.

Condition Four is the major point of connection between the Lifestyle Risk Reduction Model and the Social Development Model, notably, the resiliency part of the Model. However, Condition Four—"I want to make low-risk choices"—supports Conditions One and Two—"It could happen to me" and "I know what to do." As seen in Table 5.2, these other two models do not address Conditions One or Two. Thus, we believe the models would be strengthened by using them with the Lifestyle Risk Reduction Model. It is powerful to be bonded to a group that expects low-risk choices. It is more powerful to be bonded to such a group when people believe that these problems could happen to them, understand that only individual choices are protective, and know specifically what behaviors are low risk.

Condition Five: "I Have the Skills I Need"

People develop skills that will allow them to implement low-risk choices in their daily lives.

If people believe the problem could happen to them, know what is low risk, have strong environmental support for low-risk choices, and strong internal support, yet do not have the skills to deal with pressure to make high-risk choices, they could still end up with problems. Skill development is the final piece used to effectively promote low-risk behaviors.

Condition Five has had the most successful and intense development of any of the conditions. Thus, Lifestyle Risk Reduction practitioners can draw on a variety of sources to accomplish this condition, especially with young people. Peer resistance strategies can be used by applying curricula based on the Social Influences Model. This would include Project Smart®, Project STAR®, and Project Alert®. Curricula such as Lifeskills, based on the Personal and Social Competence Model, provide additional skill development. In addition, a variety of strategies to build resilience have come from the Social Development Model and related risk and resiliency theory. Of course, each of the above can be used separate from the Lifestyle Risk Reduction Model. The difference is that when Lifestyle Risk Reduction practitioners use these strategies, the practitioner will implement them in a way that is informed by and furthers the establishment of Condition One—"It could happen to me"—and Condition Two—"I know what to do."

PUTTING THEM ALL TOGETHER

The five principles provide a framework for establishing the conditions. The first two conditions—"It could happen to me; my choices matter" and "I know what to do"—become the core around which the other conditions revolve. Then in Conditions Three, Four, and Five, those beliefs and behaviors are supported by the environment, attitudes, values, and skills.

The conditions should generally be implemented in sequence. There are times, though, when this does not occur. Some communities are so disorganized, chaotic, and filled with danger that members of the community cannot focus on anything but staying safe, or finding food or shelter for another day. One prevention specialist told us of a conversation with an 11-year-old boy who was severely depressed subsequent to ongoing sexual abuse. The boy had been "huffing" gasoline until he passed out, even though he hated the experience. He did it because when he was passed out, he at least did not feel anything. He further exclaimed, "Those prevention people are just stupid. They come in and tell us that drugs will kill us. Don't they know we want to die?" While this young man is not typical of the prevention audience, it seems clear that any successful work with him would need to begin with Conditions Four and Five. He has to develop a desire to live, and skills to cope with his life, before anything else will make sense. People in such desperate situations couldn't care less that alcohol and drug problems could happen to them. They are not ready to hear about their quantity/frequency choices.

Currently popular, youth-focused prevention models address Conditions Three, Four, and Five very well. They alter the environment, change self-concept and develop skills. As illustrated in Table 5.2, though, none of them address Conditions One and Two, nor do they *completely* address Conditions Three, Four and Five. Of the three most popular youth-focused models, only the Social Development Model addresses Condition Three, while the Social Development and Personal and Social Skills Models have demonstrated success in addressing Conditions Four and Five.[1] By using the Lifestyle Risk Reduction Model as the guiding model for prevention, all five conditions can be addressed.

---

[1] Condition Three addresses the environment. Thus, it may seem that the Social Influences Model should address Condition Three. However, that model does not attempt to change the environment, only the person's response to the environment, which is covered in Conditions Four and Five.

SUMMARY

Alcohol and drug problems rarely occur with each episode of use. If they did, there would be very little use. In fact, the majority of times when people use alcohol or drugs, nothing bad happens, lulling the user into a false sense of security and adding to each user's belief that, "I can handle it." Addiction gradually sneaks up on the user. No one drink, one pill, or one "hit" causes the problem, yet every high-risk choice contributes to the overall problem as reflected in alcohol- and drug-related deaths, injuries, illness, and social problems.

Preventing alcohol- and drug-related problems is important and like most everything else it cannot be accomplished by just going out and doing it. It takes attention to details. Specifically, it takes attention to each high-risk choice. Behavior is the ultimate risk and protective factor, and success requires understanding that each high-risk choice is not just a single incident, but a building block of a problem. In contrast, low-risk choices are the building blocks of a life that is free of alcohol- and drug-related problems.

6

Maximizing Behavior
Change

If you would win a man to your cause—persuasion, kind,
unassuming persuasion should ever be adopted.

—Abraham Lincoln, addressing the
Washingtonian Temperance Society

If the purpose of prevention is to change human behavior, then a
shift is required in how we view ourselves and our approach. We are
not simply carrying out alcohol and drug education or other prevention activities, we are promoting behavior change. Success requires
that every decision and task is completed in a way that maximizes
this change.

Research shows that for preventive education to demonstrate
behavioral change the approach must be long enough to allow the
change process. To date, successful programs have ranged from 8 to
30 hours in length, yet prevention programs are frequently two hours
or less. It is not surprising that teachers, ministers, employers, or
others want a quick fix. They have no basis for knowing that
something different is needed. Prevention practitioners should
know. We are concerned at how often prevention practitioners agree
to do programs that are not likely to change behavior and make no
effort to negotiate the time needed to make it work. We must move
beyond defining success by how well participants like the program.

Ultimately, the only meaningful measure of success is changed behavior that leads to reduction in problems.

Of course, time itself is not what brings behavior change. To be successful we must use the time to deliver messages and activities that will change old ways of thinking, bring new insights, motivate interest in adopting new behaviors, teach new skills, allow for practice, and develop social support for the new behaviors. These things take time. To impact behavior, prevention educators must be aware of both the theory of and research on behavior change. It is easy to teach what makes people feel good instead of teaching what changes behavior. When we are working to reduce high-risk use, for example, prevention will not always "feel good." People who are making high-risk choices often "love" what those choices do for them in the short term. We are asking them to give up that short-term, tangible benefit in order to avoid a long-term problem that may or may not occur. To be successful, we need to raise enough doubt and make risk real enough to outweigh the personal short-term benefit. This is not likely to be comfortable for a person participating in the prevention program.

To accomplish this difficult task, we cannot rely on just "touching" the person either emotionally or logically. Success will require "touching" both the head and the heart, while working to systematically defuse both the belief system and the defense mechanisms that have sustained the high-risk behavior. This may sound a bit like therapy. Education that is capable of changing behavior will have a number of things in common with therapy. It certainly shares the same goals of bringing insight, provoking self-analysis, changing self-concept, empowering the person to act, and changing behavior. Such "therapeutic education" has limited focus on changing knowledge. Information becomes only a means to an end, never an end in itself. We are not trying to change what people *know*—we are trying to change what they *do*. Prevention professionals do not have to think of themselves as therapists, but the work should be thought of as a process of change and the role as being agents of change.

THE PROCESS OF PLANNED CHANGE

Lewin (1947) suggested there are three stages to the process of change. As a mental image, it may be useful to think of a block of ice that is going to be transformed into a swan statue using a mold. The first step in the process of this change is unfreezing. This requires time, patience, and the proper environment. The second stage is the change itself. This happens rapidly as the melted water is poured into the mold. Though the change happens rapidly, it is not stable until the third stage, refreezing, occurs. This last stage requires time and the proper environment. Applying Lewin's stages of change to prevention is enlightening.

Unfreezing Stage

We often pursue change too quickly. Just as an organic gardener first works to feed the soil before planting, the change agent works first to unfreeze—to warm the person to the possibility of change. This phase may take 40 percent to 50 percent of the time involved in the change process and how we approach this phase is critical. Lewin (1973) conceptualized this process in terms of a "force field analysis" which allows the change agent to analyze the forces working for and against change (see Fig. 6.1). To conduct a force field analysis, draw a vertical line down the center of a page. This represents the status quo of the person (community or group). In other words, it represents the behavior that we want to change. For the sake of our illustration, the left side of the paper represents the direction of high-risk behaviors and the right side represents low-risk behaviors. We want to move the person's behavior (status quo line) toward the low-risk behaviors—the right side. The per-

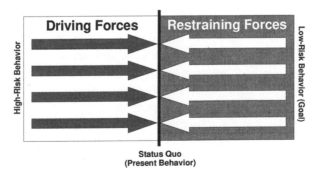

Figure 6.1.   Force field analysis.

son's behavior is what it is for a variety of reasons: beliefs, attitudes, personality traits, biological responses, peer influences, family influences, and perceived benefits of use that promote the behavior. These are the "restraining forces." They restrain change which keeps behavior from changing in the desired direction. On the other side of the line are a variety of "driving forces" that are actually promoting low-risk choices. These might include laws, costs, perception of risks, personality, job, friends, family, or religious beliefs. When using this approach for a particular person or group, it is important to identify, as specifically as possible, exact beliefs, attitudes, people, or perceptions that influence behavior positively or negatively.

After identifying the driving and restraining forces, a plan can be made for altering the forces and, ultimately, the behavior. In general, the status quo line will move all by itself if we are successful in either: (1) weakening or removing restraining forces; (2) adding or strengthening driving forces; or (3) redirecting restraining forces into driving forces.

People commonly add driving forces by applying pressure, encouragement, or inducement to change the behavior. Our natural tendency is to "go in with big guns," scaring, reasoning, encouraging with slogans, cajoling, appealing to the law or authority, or otherwise trying to "push" people in the desired direction, yet this is generally the least successful approach to unfreezing. We illustrate this in training settings by asking two participants to hold a book between them. One person represents driving forces, the other restraining forces. While they are exerting equal pressure the book remains at status quo, balanced between the two forces. Then we ask the person representing driving forces to push and the other person to do whatever comes naturally. Almost without exception when the first person increases pressure, the second person instinctively pushes back. That is often what happens with individuals and communities when we attempt to move the status quo with driving forces. It can provoke opposition. Instead, our energy is usually better spent on removing restraining forces. When we remove the support for the high-risk choices, the status quo will move with less effort.

This is not unlike the story of the contest between the sun and the wind. The wind had seen a man who was walking down the street wearing a coat and challenged the sun to see who could make him remove his coat. The wind went first, blowing with all its might attempting to blow the coat off the man's back. But the stronger the wind blew, the more tightly the man held to his coat, wrapping it around himself. When the wind stopped, the sun then turned on the warmth and shone down on the man. After a while, the man removed the coat himself. A successful unfreezing stage will generally be more like the sun than the wind, using light and warmth as tools to promote change.

Having said that, we also add a caution against "feel good" prevention. Emotions have too often been traded for reliable information. It does not seem likely that any number of "I'm Special" buttons, cute songs, or "warm fuzzies" used alone are going to prevent alcohol and drug problems. When we say "light and warmth," we mean a nonjudgmental approach that is enlightened and enlightening, aimed at very specific restraining forces.

As noted earlier, Bachman el al.'s (1988) analysis of *Monitoring the Future* data reported that low perception of risk preceded increased use. Increasing perception of risk associated with high-risk behaviors will reduce that restraining force. Successfully changing attitudes which are predictive of behavior removes another driving force for high-risk choices. Perkins and Berkowitz (1986) and Haines and Spear (1996) reported that misperceptions of the norm, believing that more use is occurring than is reality encourages use; correcting these perceptions reduces use. These are examples of very specific forces that prevention can target in the unfreezing stage. We often attempt to move too quickly in prevention. Only when we complete the unfreezing stage can we effectively begin to promote the desired behavior. This takes time.

Change Stage

If the unfreezing stage is completed properly, the change falls from the tree like a ripe apple. Although a great struggle can precede change, most of that is part of the unfreezing. Once the person decides to change, the process is only half completed. If the process is not completed, people are likely to return to their previous behaviors. The new behavior needs time to become established and incorporated into everyday life.

Refreezing Stage

It is estimated that the unfreezing stage takes about 40 to 50 percent of the time and effort in the change process, and the refreezing stage takes another 40 to 45 percent. This is the time of stabilizing the change, including building ongoing commitment to a low-risk lifestyle and developing personal and interpersonal skills needed to maintain a low-risk lifestyle. People have to first believe, then experience, that they can find pleasure, success, and satisfaction in life without relying on high-risk choices. This is true for both the young person, who has never used drugs or alcohol, and the adult, who is struggling to give up high-risk choices.

In the Five Conditions of the Lifestyle Risk Reduction Model, the unfreezing stage occurs primarily when establishing Conditions One and Two, though some also occurs in establishing Conditions Three and Four. Change itself occurs sometime after establishing the first two conditions, and the refreezing stage occurs while establishing Conditions Three, Four, and Five. By mentally superimposing the stages of change over the five conditions, each takes on a three-dimensional quality. Assisting people as they move through the conditions and the three phases of change requires attention to what is done, as well as to how it is done. To explain how it is being done, it is useful to draw on findings from persuasion research.

PERSUASION: "KIND, UNASSUMING PERSUASION"

Lincoln's words to the Washingtonian Temperance Society were decades ahead of the first research on the topic of persuasive communication (see Box 6.1), yet his words summarize most of what research validates. There is, indeed, a "road to (people's) reason," and, unintentionally, we can cause them to "retreat within themselves and close all doors." Young adults in particular report that they are turned off by prevention programs that they believe attempt to control their lives. It is difficult, but important, to guide people to the desired behavior without making them feel that their freedom to choose is not respected, or that their lives are controlled.

As one young man said, "If just once you had tried to control us or tell us what we had to do, I would have had every reason I needed to ignore everything you were saying. But you didn't do that, and now it (the message) is in my head and my heart, and I have to do something about it." There can be a thin line between expressing deep concern and the desire to help (initiating appreciation of the message) and expressing judgment and desire to control (provoking rejection of the message). If people are to be convinced about prevention, prevention presentation is incredibly important. Kind, unassuming persuasion fills this need.

If there are cardinal rules of persuasion they would probably be: (1) know where your audience is in their attitudes, beliefs, and behaviors; (2) structure messages to meet the audience where they are and take them where you want them to go; (3) present the message in a credible way; and (4) avoid provoking defenses.

Box 6.1.
From Lincoln's Address to the
Washingtonian Temperance Society, 1842

When the conduct of men is designed to be influenced, persuasion, kind, unassuming persuasion should ever be adopted. . . . If you would win a man to your cause, first convince him you are his sincere friend. Therein is a drop of honey that catches his heart; which, say what he will, is the high road to his reason, and which, once gained, you will find but little trouble in convincing his judgment of the justice of your cause, if indeed it is a just cause. On the contrary, attempt to dictate to his judgment, or to command his action, or to mark him as one to be shunned and despised, and he will retreat within himself, close all avenues to his head and his heart, and though your cause be naked truth itself, transformed to the heaviest steel. . . . You will no more be able to pierce him, than to penetrate the hard shell of a tortoise with a rye-straw. Such is man, and so must he be understood by those who would lead him, event to his own best interests.

First Cardinal Rule—Know Where Your Audience Is in Their Attitudes, Beliefs, and Behaviors

Advertisers spend hundreds of millions of dollars each year for research because they know the importance of knowing their audience. It is no less important for prevention. Important questions need to be asked: "What barriers will the audience have to hearing this message?"; "How will this message conflict with their perceptions of reality?"; "What forces in their lives encourage low-risk choices that I can build on?"; "What do they want more than high-risk choices that high-risk choices will jeopardize?"; "Will this message move them closer to adopting the desired behaviors?"; and "Is this message effective in changing one of the restraining forces behind high-risk choices?" Whenever the reality of the prevention audience makes the prevention message impossible to hear or act on, there must always be an accommodation in how—or whether—a prevention message is presented.

Prevention fundamentals will not change. Low risk is low risk; high risk is high risk; it is always biology plus quantity and frequency, rather than the kind of person, that increases risk for problems. These things do not change just because the audience wants them not to be true. But how is the topic approached so that it will be heard, accepted, and acted on? We may speak the wisdom of the ages, but if the audience cannot hear, accept, and act on it, we might as well have said nothing.

At this point, universal needs are safely targeted in broad prevention messages. For instance, most people believe that alcoholism represents some form of personal weakness and that personal strength is more important than drinking choices in preventing alcoholism. Given this, it makes sense to work on undoing that belief. Other driving forces, such as social support for high-risk drinking, are unique to a group and prevention programs must be specifically tailored to promote change.

The core concepts in our message do not change; the only change is the way in which the message is presented. Judgments must always be made about which messages are important. The important issue is whether the message moves a person closer to adopting prevention behaviors. If a message is clear, and delivering it has a good "feel," but the message creates a barrier to the ultimate adoption of a prevention goal, then it should be changed. For example, both parents and children can become confused when prevention messages emphasize that alcohol is a drug, without helping them understand and make sense of the legal differences (see Chapter 2).

Effective prevention calls on us to question our assumptions. Is there any evidence that simply knowing "alcohol is a drug" discourages the use of alcohol? There is evidence that Lifestyle Risk Reduction curricula can increase abstinence and reduce high-risk drinking without mentioning that alcohol is a drug. If a program is going to stress that alcohol is a drug, how can we change our discussion to make sense of the legality for adults so that we remove the problems that the message sometimes creates? For example, it seems likely that the message is least helpful when comparing alcohol to illegal drugs. Instead, the prevention program could stress that, in addition to illegal drugs, there are a wide variety of legal drugs which vary in risk. These include medicinal drugs—both over-the-counter medications and prescription drugs—as well as nonmedicinal drugs, such as caffeine, nicotine, and alcohol. Medicinal drugs come with directions for use which need to be strictly followed to reduce risk. Nonmedicinal, legal drugs do not come with directions for use, but the need to manage risk is great for those who choose to use these substances. Risk is especially great for nicotine and alcohol. The program can then provide guidelines to manage risk (see discussion of guidelines in Chapter 5). In this way, we make the point that alcohol is a drug without confusing legal and illegal drugs.

Effective prevention also calls on us to examine our motives. In our experience, some people use "alcohol is a drug," or other favorite phrases, somewhat like a hammer. It is important for us to distinguish between delivering a message to meet the needs of our audience, and delivering a message to meet our own emotional needs.

Effective prevention challenges us to find what is meaningful to them, not to us. For example, when working with illegal drug users, teens who drink, and DUI offenders, education programs often emphasize the law. There is no doubt that laws can discourage high-risk behaviors. Either fear of, or respect for, the law is a major reason why many people do not use illegal drugs, drink as teens, or drive impaired. Therefore, emphasizing the law to people who have not yet engaged in those behaviors may reduce the number who ever will do so. However, few people who violate these laws are unaware of the law. Teens who drink know it is illegal. People who drink and drive know it is illegal. Legal knowledge is not enough to deter them. The experience of getting caught may well be a deterrence to future violations. However, will an educational program that emphasizes the law make a difference for people who have demonstrated disregard for the law? Not likely. It is often hard for law-abiding citizens to realize how little meaning the law has to some individuals. Rather than assuming the audience values what we value, we need to know more about them. What does this audience value that their high-risk behavior is jeopardizing? Perhaps an arrest will take away their money, their freedom, or their driver's license. The law may not matter, but these things might. What will make the risks real to that person?

On the other hand, there are times when we have more in common with our audience than we think. Some prevention workers routinely ignore speeding laws, but are appalled that others ignore drinking age laws or drinking-driving laws. Those of us who speed are not ignorant of the speeding laws. We simply do not value those laws as highly as we value our time. We have convinced ourselves that speeding laws are minor and of little importance. We also do not really believe that our speeding is going to kill us or other people. We have heard the data on how each extra five miles per hour increases risk for crash and death, we just don't think it will happen to us. We may get caught, but we are willing to take that risk. It may be useful to realize that we all are using similar defense mechanisms to justify our behavior. Some people use those defenses for drinking, others for speeding. We need to meet people where they are and address the reality of their lives. Sometimes we can do this by being more in touch with the reality of our own lives.

Second Cardinal Rule—Structure the Message to Meet the Audience Where They Are and Take Them Where You Want Them to Go

Once we know where people are and what is meaningful to them, messages must be structured to take them where we want them to go. This is both a content and a process issue.

The search for the most effective and useful content for preventive education has been ongoing for at least three decades. Research in the 1960s and early 1970s (Ellickson & Robyn, 1987; Falck & Craig, 1988) reported that no available alcohol and drug education programs had demonstrated a positive impact on behavior; some even spurred an increase in use following the education. In addition, research demonstrated that the more people knew about drugs, the more they used or, perhaps conversely, the more people used drugs, the more they learned about drugs. Some concluded that drug education could be harmful. The federal government at that time called for a moratorium on drug-specific education and the emphasis shifted to affective education aimed at increasing self-esteem and interpersonal skills (Vicary, 1979). But research on affective education also reported little positive impact on drug use, with some studies revealing an increase in use following affective education.

At this point, there seems to be little reason to believe that either teaching general facts about drugs or teaching general skills will have an impact on drug use behavior. But neither is there reason to despair. There are now several curricula that have demonstrated an impact on behavior, and we can learn from their success. We now know that content must be tailored to each individual and to the specific behavior we want to change. Unfortunately, most prevention programs reflect approaches that have not worked. Let's first concentrate on alcohol- and drug-specific content.

A shift in prevention activities must be made from changing knowledge to changing behavior. When the goal is to change knowledge, available knowledge will be used to target knowledgeable change for the age and experience of the audience. The starting and ending point is the knowledge. When the goal is to change behavior, the desired behavioral outcome is the focus. Before starting, the specific behaviors for change are identified. In keeping with our earlier discussion of prevention goals, it is not enough to simply say, "The goal is no use or zero tolerance." To be most effective, the target is increasing abstinence, delaying onset of use, and reducing high-risk use. High risk and low risk must be clearly defined, as was done in Chapter 5. From this definition, a force field analysis can be carried out to identify the specific beliefs, attitudes, and other forces that are driving and restraining change. For example, prior to developing any Lifestyle Risk Reduction curricula, Prevention Research Institute identified specific attitudes that correlated with low-risk and high-risk choices. Van Tubergen, Daugherty, O'Bryan and Morrow (unpublished research) conducted a Q-sort analysis that identified attitude patterns which were conceptualized as prevailing beliefs that could be targeted. The Q-sort items were based on the earlier referenced attitude research that had been done by Daugherty and Thompson (unpublished research) and tested by Carver (1982). The strongest belief pattern was that alcohol problems happened because of some personal weakness. Conversely, these problems are prevented by personal strength. This view also included an element of pleasure; that, at least for the person who "knows how to handle it," drinking is fun. The second view was that alcohol problems are willful, self-inflicted, and can be avoided if a person just wants to. This view also contains an element of strength—specifically, strength of character. The third view was that alcoholism was caused by heredity: People are either born with it, or they could never develop it. The perception that drinking problems are caused by something other than drinking is common to all of these beliefs. These views appear to be driving forces behind high-risk drinking. They also are amenable to change. Thus, the program authors *carefully selected* content that seemed relevant and useful for changing these forces (Daugherty & O'Bryan, 1986, 1996). As previously noted, later research indicates that changes in these beliefs correlate with reductions in high-risk drinking and reductions in recidivism (Thompson, 1996).

We believe that there is no place for "everything you wanted to know about drugs" in a persuasive approach to preventive education. What a person wants to know and what we want them to know is virtually irrelevant. The most important thing is what will help weaken or remove the driving force, strengthen a restraining force, and encourage adoption of the behavior.

Persuasive messages must be carefully crafted. Jean Kilbourne (1991), a media analyst and critic, points out that every detail of an advertisement is carefully planned, designed, placed, airbrushed, and tweaked, as well as tested for maximum impact. To the extent possible, this should be done for prevention, as illustrated by the process described above. Although the multimillion dollar budgets that alcohol advertisers have are not available to prevention, the capability is available to apply careful thought, consideration, preparation, testing, revision, and improvement to grow the most powerful prevention programs possible.[1]

When the most appropriate and powerful content is gathered and the target for the prevention is identified, the persuasion process must be addressed. Most traditional teaching methods are designed to change what people know. Persuasion is designed to change what people believe and do. One of the most helpful persuasion techniques we have found is McGuire's persuasion process (1947). There are two "versions" of this process. The first version is used when the audience is not likely to agree with the position being promoted; there are four steps in this process.

Step One—Identify the View that You Want to Change

Attitudes, beliefs, and assumptions are often unconscious. While prevention information should be persuasive, we have no certainty that the audience will make a link between that information and the "view" we are hoping to change. By verbalizing a view, it is brought to consciousness so the audience cannot help but mentally

---

[1] One of the things that has worked against this approach is prevention fads. The approach vacillates from "Just Say No" Clubs to Red Ribbon Campaigns to the curriculum *du jour*. Another issue is the turnover in the people who are carrying out prevention. Many community prevention programs have different staff every one to two years. Prevention programs may be better served to double salaries for half as many staff whom they could retain four times as long. Expertise takes time. Thus, fads and turnover are major issues.

compare it with the information we present. It is important to the change process for the "view" to be verbalized before any effort is made to change it. We can state it ourselves, or it can be processed and "drawn out" of the audience. If we "draw" it from the audience, there are important steps to take to guard against provoking defenses. We will explain that process below when we address the fourth cardinal rule—avoid provoking defenses.

Step Two—Validate the Reasonableness of the View that You Want to Change

After the view targeted for change has been drawn out or stated, it is important to validate its reasonableness. Note that we are not validating the accuracy, but the reasonableness. This process should not be long and detailed, as we do not wish to reinforce the view, but neither should this step be halfhearted. No matter how incorrect a point of view, it is valid to the person who holds it. When we first acknowledge the reasonableness without discounting the view, the audience feels understood and is more receptive to listening further. If we skip this step, it is likely to come up in the audience's mind as a "yes, but" after we present our information. By stating the point-of-view first, our argument is framed in terms of their belief, and removes much of its "power" as a rebuttal. In these first two steps, it is important to avoid statements that would imply that the view we want to change is incorrect, since it may be a commonly held view that seems reasonable. It is not a myth; it is not wrong; it is not even a misperception for people holding the view. Without drawing any conclusion about the accuracy of the point of view, the audience is invited to explore its "accuracy."

Step Three—Challenge the View with New Information

Having completed Steps One and Two, it is time to present new information. It may be new to the audience or it may be information they have heard before, but presented in a way that gives it new meaning. In either case, the goal is for the person to experience, "I have always believed 'the view' and I wasn't silly for believing it. I sure didn't know this new information; maybe I need to reconsider." For example, consider an audience that believes alcoholism is caused by heredity and, thus, cannot be prevented. The implication is that drinking choices are irrelevant as a cause or prevention of alcoholism. To challenge this, the prevention worker can walk the audience through the logic of twin research as described in Chapter 3. Then the leader can ask the audience to identify what twin research would show if alcoholism is controlled by heredity. They would answer that if one identical twin developed alcoholism, the other twin would develop alcoholism 100 percent of the time. Then they can discover that research shows that identical twins do not have the same concordance rate. In fact, the second twin develops alcoholism 50 percent of the time or less. People who came into this activity believing that alcoholism is controlled by heredity are moved toward letting go of that belief. This would be one step in a long process of undoing old ways of thinking and establishing new beliefs—that is, a process of moving from the belief "alcoholism is caused by heredity," to the belief "heredity establishes a level of risk and alcoholism is triggered by quantity and frequency of drinking." It is important to keep in mind that the information—not the presenter—is doing the challenging. And the view is being challenged, not the audience. This is meant to be "kind, unassuming persuasion."

Step Four—Replace the Old View with a New View

McGuire points out that even after giving the same information to a number of people, they are likely to draw a number of different conclusions. We cannot assume that the audience will draw the conclusion we want them to make. If we do a good job with the first three steps, then the audience should be prepared for Step Four and be receptive to the message. Some will say, "Yeah, that's what I was just thinking." However, for the majority the experience will be, "That makes sense, I understand things in a new way now." If we are not getting something close to those two responses from most of the audience, then we need to go back and redesign the presentation. According to McGuire, this approach is more likely to change beliefs, and to inoculate, making it less likely that people will revert to their old point of view at a later time.

When the Audience Already Agrees

Younger audiences are frequently most receptive to alcohol and drug prevention. Most fourth-graders say that alcohol and drugs are bad and they never want to use them. By high school, a majority have used alcohol and/or drugs. Between these ages, they need an inoculation against changing their view. McGuire (1947) suggests that this can be done with a different sequence:

1. State the view that the audience holds and that you want to encourage.
2. Give information to support the view.
3. State the view that they will face in the future and that you wish to inoculate against.
4. Give the reasonableness of that view.
5. State the view they already hold and why it is a more accurate view.

A person who was exposed to this approach prior to being introduced to the "opposing view" is likely to have a response of, "I've heard that before and here is why that is not correct." Prevention Research Institute has been using McGuire's process as an outline for prevention education since 1982. In our experience, most audiences respond best to his original four step process. However, curricula for elementary age students should use the five step modified process.

Other Persuasion Techniques that Help Move People to a New View

McGuire's persuasion process has been the most helpful approach in our work, but we have found several other approaches also to be useful:

Engagement. In order for persuasion to be successful, it is essential to interactively engage participants in the change process. If a particular belief is the target for change, that belief will be made conscious for participants and either internally (within the person) or externally (within the group) will become part of the participants' process as they struggle with the new information. Engagement is likely to be most effective when it is multilevel, involving the person emotionally and intellectually.

Interactivity is key to the engagement process. For example, Tobler and Stratton's (1997) metaanalysis of prevention effectiveness showed that the interactive peer resistance programs are effective, while noninteractive peer resistance programs are not. However, simply making a program interactive does not necessarily make it engaging, or increase the likelihood of behavior change. Affective education programs are often very interactive, but do not appear to change drug use. Interactivity can be purely external, but engagement will always be internal. For example, lectures can be engaging with the integration of persuasion processes. Engagement is used to capture the attention and involvement of the participant with an attitude, belief, skill, or targeted behavior. Successful engagement, at some point, becomes affective without the need for the simulation that is common in affective education.

Creating Cognitive Dissonance. Raising doubt is one of the most powerful tools for initiating behavior change. People do not change if they are comfortable. A certain amount of anxiety and healthy questions about whether our views are accurate, and whether our behaviors will hurt, is helpful in initiating change. Sometimes it is better to leave a person with a question than with an answer, at least for a period of time. Perhaps this is one of the strengths of the first three steps of McGuire's persuasion process. Identifying the view and laying it side by side with new information that challenges it creates cognitive dissonance when both statements cannot be true. The fourth step in the process provides the way out of the dissonance.

Group Consensus. When a group discusses an issue and comes to consensus, the tendency for group members is to defend that consensus. However, consensus should not be introduced early in a prevention program because the group can reach a very different agreement than the desired prevention goals. In other words, group consensus should not be used until basic concepts have been discussed and the group leader is comfortable that the group will come to consensus in the desired direction. Otherwise, moving the group to a more "prevention compatible" position will be more difficult. In a design for success, the group discussion should not be too open-ended.

Rhetorical Questions. Years ago, Salem cigarettes had a television and radio advertisement that included the jingle, "You can take Salem out of the country but—you can't take the country out of Salem." After some time of airing, the ad's catchy tune changed to stop immediately after the word, "but—." The listener could not help it—the end of the jingle, "you can't take the country out of Salem" would play over and over again in the listener's mind. It was a very clever use of the principle of rhetorical questions.

A rhetorical question is one that does not need to be answered because everyone knows the answer. Because the answer is known, it will immediately come to mind as soon as it is asked. "In what month is Christmas?" When you read the question, you can't keep "December" out of your mind. One application of using rhetorical questions in prevention is to take a key point and word it as a question at a point that people might have figured out the answer. If no one answers, give the answer. But at logical places in the presentation, keep coming back to the question. After the first time, people will not be able to keep the answer from coming to mind, and it slowly becomes theirs.

Repetition. It may irritate you that the same television ad plays several times in the same program, but it is not easily forgotten. It has been said that a fact must be repeated more than a dozen times before everyone in the group has heard it, let alone remembers it. While too much repetition can become counterproductive, a certain amount of repetition is vital to the persuasion process.

In our own work we apply this principle by repeatedly bringing the audience back to one or two primary conclusions. For example, we sequence the material to come back repeatedly and logically to the question, "Who can develop alcoholism?" To which the audience learns to respond, "Anyone!" With repetition, participants come to hear the answer in their mind before they say the words. The words, though, are now coming from participants instead of the group leader. As one participant wrote, "It was pounded into our heads, but by the end of the class I was beginning to believe it. Who could develop alcoholism? Anyone—and that meant me!"

The above principles represent only a sampling of the persuasion principles that can help implement the second cardinal rule—"Structure the message to meet the audience where they are and take them where you want them to go."

After carefully choosing the content of the message and structuring its delivery to reflect persuasion, there are two additional cardinal rules for persuasion to be effective.

Third Cardinal Rule—Present the Message with Credibility

Credibility is multifaceted. The information in the message must be credible. One of the difficulties prevention faces with adults and young adults is that they are skeptical because they feel they have received prevention messages that are emotional overstatements. This skepticism must be overcome before progress can be made.

Alcohol and drug education messages have become more credible in the past two decades. We would like to think that the days of *Reefer Madness* are behind us, but we still struggle with putting impact over accuracy. For example, in the 1980s, there was much talk that teens developed alcoholism more quickly than adults because their hypothalamus was not fully developed. We searched for the source of this message and any research supporting the claim. We finally traced it to a book written by a physician at a Veterans Administration hospital (Valles, 1969) who, in one paragraph, wondered whether such a thing might possibly be true. It seems his wondering turned into fact as it passed from person to person.

Similarly, we still find numerous prevention messages which indicate "while it takes years for an adult to develop alcoholism, teens develop alcoholism in as little as six months." We wonder what the source of that statement is and what evidence verifies it. We have searched for research and have not found it, although we have found research that appears to challenge it. For example, the reader may recall earlier references to research showing that people who develop alcoholism, on the average, initiate drinking at an older age than their peers (Goodwin et al., 1973; Plaut, 1967), and research that indicates that age of first use was significant only in those with a family history of alcoholism (Kubicka et al., 1990). We contacted the publishers of this claim and have found no scientific support, other than the impression that teens in treatment for addiction had a rapid course of addiction. Obviously, anything that happens to teens develops rather quickly. Teens who develop cancer develop it with fewer years of living than adults who develop cancer. Does this mean that teens develop cancer more quickly? We discussed this issue in Chapter 1.

What happens to credibility when teens receive this information and then notice some years later that most of the people they know have been drinking longer than six months without developing alcoholism? The unfortunate tendency is to discount everything that comes from that source. It is very important to be accurate with prevention messages. Mistakes are made and new research modifies information; these things are inevitable. But when we hear something we like at a conference, don't check its validity, then make it a central point of our approach, we are on thin ice. The more central any point is to our message, and the more remarkable the point, the greater the need to check the original source and verify that there is enough data to support the point.

We could develop a rather troubling list of frequently cited alcohol and drug "facts" that appear to have no grounding in research. We find it useful to have the scientific references easily available for anything we teach. We would suggest that people who use "packaged" prevention materials should require reference documentation of the developer; those who develop their own materials should include references. The prevention professional does not need to have personally read each of the several hundred studies that might support the content of a curriculum, but the presenter should be able to produce references when asked. Simply put, we need to do everything possible to ensure that content has credibility.

This is another area that comes into much sharper focus with young adults and adults. Children have little basis for questioning what they are being taught—at least at a young age. However, young adults and adults who have had more experience with drugs and alcohol must receive messages that ring true to their experience. There is no room for overstatement.

Credibility is also related to the presenter. Sometimes people are credible because of the position they have, what they have accomplished, or what they have experienced. One survey (LoBello, Tarpley, & Day, 1988) with teens asked them to rate the credibility of 22 possible sources of alcohol information. The findings were enlightening. The number one source of credible information was their own experience. It is important always to keep in mind that this is the major competition for any prevention message. Interestingly, the second most credible source of information was recovering people, followed closely by parents, ministers, police officers, and doctors, in that order. The least credible sources were friends who drink, movie/TV stars, active alcoholics, television, newspapers, professional athletes, nondrinking friends, and social workers. Teachers were right in the middle. It is interesting that the sources prevention programs use most often were rated the least credible. This should raise questions about the broadly held assumptions that peer programs, television ads, and role models, such as athletes and movie stars, are credible sources. It would also appear that the value of parents in prevention, as well as ministers, doctors, and police officers, is underrated and underused.

Credible sources, combined with credible relevance and per-suasively delivered messages, should provide the greatest impact. When giving the message, close attention should be given to staying consistent with the criteria described above. For example, people recovering from heart attacks do not "tell their story" as a prevention approach; instead they would talk about "how to prevent what happened to me." In the same way, a straight "AA lead" (telling one's story) is important for an Alcoholics Anonymous meeting, or for an intervention program with people who may have alcoholism, but is questionable when used as a prevention message. However, a recov-ering person saying, "These are the beliefs I held that made me feel my drinking choices did not matter; this is what I have learned since; and this is what you can do to prevent the development of this health problem" might be effective.

We do not have to be Nobel prize winners to be credible, or even be in one of the categories listed above in order to be effective.

Presenters who are well prepared, articulate, and confident project credibility. They give the audience a sense that "this person knows."

Audiences also tend to assign greater credibility to people that they perceive as being like them and who are likable. Unfortunately, prevention workers often make presentations to groups they may not like. If we do not like an audience, they are not prone to find us a credible source. Our discounting of them comes through and is returned to us. There is something interesting, something likable in every group of people. We do not have to approve of their lifestyles or enjoy their personalities. But we do need to find that point of connection and appreciation of them or there is no basis for credibility and human connection. Lincoln's words again ring true, "First convince him you are his sincere friend." This requires communicating nonjudgment, acceptance, and a *nonverbal* sense of "I like you; I'm glad to be here with you."

Finally, individuals not only assign credibility to people they like and feel like them, they also assign credibility to people they perceive as having something in common with them. This does not require being part of a group or having external connections. It cannot be bought in any lasting way by emphasizing some surface connection. It must be demonstrated. Words and actions must show that we understand our audience's reality and do not judge it. For example, we have heard prevention professionals say to heavy drinkers, "I don't know why anyone would want to get drunk. You just end up with your head in the toilet." Everyone who loves to get drunk immediately experiences, "This person is not like us; this person does not know what it is all about." Contrast this with another group where a participant said, "People would like it a lot better if you said 0–8 drinks is low risk." The presenter immediately responded, "Of course they would. It would be a lot more fun. But, unfortunately low risk is not determined by what makes us happy, but by research on what creates risk." That response met the person where he was (drinking is fun) and took him where he needed to go (8 drinks is always high risk) and was done in a way that the person could experience, "This presenter knows what it is all about." Such a response builds trust.

This way of responding is another benefit of McGuire's persuasion process. When we successfully identify what people believe, and do a credible job of stating why that view makes sense to them, then we have essentially demonstrated to them that we are on their wavelength and why. This is often enough to establish credibility.

Carefully constructing the message to address the force and the desired behaviors, constructing the message to reflect the persuasion process, and paying attention to establishing credibility for both the message and the messenger, we are now close to having a high impact presentation. The success of the implementation now hinges on how well we navigate the minefields of defenses.

Fourth Cardinal Rule—Avoid Provoking Defenses

Defense mechanisms are unconscious and automatic psychological reactions that protect each of us from experiencing feelings that are threatening. We use these defenses unconsciously when we are embarrassed, when we experience loss, or when we are frightened. Defenses keep us from experiencing the full impact of these emotions. They work so well, in fact, that they can stop the change process in its tracks. This substantial defense system surrounds high-risk alcohol and drug choices and, if we provoke these defenses, the practice of change stops. The window that opened to considering change closes, at least for a period of time. However, we can adopt an attitude and learn skills that will help us navigate this minefield successfully.

One of the most important attitudes to adopt, especially when working with rebellious people or with all people who are making high-risk choices, is somewhat of a paradox. The paradox is this: *If we want to maximize the likelihood that the person will adopt the low-risk choices that we promote, then we must be perfectly willing for them to reject everything we say and continue making high-risk choices.* If we are not willing for them to reject our message, we are likely to push too hard and, as we discussed in the force field analysis, they will push back.

This is not to say that we should be indifferent. On the contrary, if we have passion for the message, passion for prevention, passion for behavior change, and passion for low-risk choices, our cause is enhanced—but only if we can teach with detachment. Only then can the person experience, "You care so much and yet you are not trying to control me." It is a lesson learned long ago by Al-Anon. If our passion for the change translates into control, when it reaches the ears and the heart of the person, we will have provoked defenses and, perhaps, rebelliousness. We will lose and they will lose. On the other hand, if they *experience* us as relating to them in a respectful way that shows that we fully accept the reality (and it is a reality) that the choice to adopt high-risk or low-risk behaviors is theirs and theirs alone, then we make it possible for them to consider the possibility of not making high-risk choices.

This is not an issue of rights. We are not saying a person has the right to make high-risk choices. In fact, given the harm that an individual's high-risk choices can inflict on innocent family members and even bystanders, a good case could be made that no one has the right to make high-risk choices of any type. For example, no one has a right to drive 100 miles per hour. But everyone who drives has that choice. This is a matter of reality. Even though the behavior may be illegal, harmful, dangerous, inconsiderate, or a violation of other people's rights, no one can take away from another person the option to choose. Our only power is the power of influence, not control. The issue for a prevention professional is: How can I become the most powerful influence possible without attempting to control the behaviors of my audience? When I slip from influence to control, I provoke defenses in my audience.

This is especially easy to confuse when working with children and adolescents. A strong message of zero-tolerance prevention is we should not give teens a choice about alcohol or drug use—as though it was ours to give or take. Imagine that we have offered you a stick of chewing gum. Having the opportunity to take the gum, is it now possible for you to not make a choice? You could take it—that's a choice. You could reject it—that's a choice. You could turn your back and ignore the offer—but that is also a choice. Even the act of not choosing is a choice. Once we have an opportunity, we must make a choice. Now think about this: Do young people in the United States have opportunities to drink or use drugs? Certainly they do. Is it possible for them not to choose or for us to remove that choice?

We think not. What caring educators have struggled with is really permission. We can give or withhold our permission for a particular choice; we cannot take away the choice. We do not have that power.

This is an important recognition for parents, teachers, and others who work with children and young people. If we think we can remove their choice, then we see little need to prepare them for making a choice. When we recognize that we cannot remove their choice, then it is evident that we need both to withhold that permission and to prepare them well for the choices they will face. There is no mixed message if it is done properly. We are not saying, "Here is what I expect, but I don't think you will do it, so . . ." Instead we are saying, "Here is what I expect. I believe you will want to do it, but it seems inevitable that you will get pressure to do something different. Let's prepare for that pressure."

Peer resistance skills training has been an important part of preparing young people for the choices they face. One of the underlying assumptions of peer resistance training, however, is that it is being taught at a time in kids' lives when most young people do not want to use—the 4th, 5th or 6th grades. By the time these children reach high school, the impact of peer resistance training seems to wear off (Hansen, 1990). People who define prevention as preventing use, and reject any goal other than total abstinence, sometimes conclude that peer resistance is a failed approach because it only works for a period of time. This has led some people to abandon the approach. That is a mistake. Peer resistance training can work well in delaying the onset of use. Once we broaden our thinking to include delaying the onset as a legitimate prevention goal, then peer resistance is an appropriate approach for that window of time. It also gives skills that people need to carry out their intention not to use. If they change their minds and want to use (as happens for most youth with alcohol), then they need a different strategy to impact what they want to do. It is at this time that we find Lifestyle Risk Reduction education to be important.

This also brings us back to the final cardinal rule of persuasion. Whether we are talking about prevention with young people who are not yet making high-risk choices, or with adults or young adults who are already making high-risk choices, it is important that we deliver our prevention message without provoking defenses or rebellion. In addition to adopting an attitude that is noncontrolling and projects respect, there are other techniques to avoid provoking defenses.

One technique is to ask questions that do not incorporate responses that include personal views or opinions. It is a widely accepted teaching technique to include participants in the learning experience by asking questions. When our goal is to teach facts, that may be fine. If the question is "What is 2 + 2?" and I don't know the answer, I might be embarrassed, but the answer is not debatable and someday I will probably learn it. There was no agenda beyond learning the information. However, when our information is being used to change attitudes, beliefs, and behaviors, we must be careful. If the teacher or group leader asks participants to share their view, or to state what they think about a particular point, and then proceeds to show how the participant's response was incorrect, that person and others in the group are likely to feel defensive and shut down. At that point it does not matter if the group leader is correct. The fact is not likely to penetrate the participants' defenses.

Instead, accomplishing the first three steps of McGuire's persuasion process needs to be kept at arm's length from the participants' ego. In drawing out the point of view we are challenging, we never ask, "What do you think?" Instead we ask, "What would *most* people say?" or we frame it in terms of the belief that we want to challenge: "If this view is true, what would we expect this research to show?"

It is also important that we use words that are not likely to carry even subtle judgment to the listener or reader. It is tempting, for example, to describe drug use or heavy drinking as being bad choices, wrong choices, or unhealthy choices. But the person who is making these choices may experience each of these words as a judgment, and when people feel judged they become defensive and less likely to change. We find that most people can hear the terms low risk and high risk without experiencing judgment. Small changes in other wording can also make a difference. When we talk with the public, we try to avoid use of the word "alcoholic," or phrases like "becoming an alcoholic." Instead, we talk about "people with alcoholism," "developing alcoholism," or "triggering alcoholism." People frequently comment on how different it sounds and feels to them. Not only does it seem less labeling and less judgmental, it also sounds more like the way most other health problems are discussed: "people with heart disease," or "people who develop cancer."

In our prevention efforts, we have abandoned any reference to alcoholism being a disease, not because we do not accept it as a disease, but because in persuasion, our point of view is not important. The point of view of the audience counts, and many people have an emotional reaction against the thought that alcoholism is a disease. In addition, people do not have to accept alcoholism as a disease in order to adopt low-risk choices. This is similar to our earlier point about alcohol being a drug. People do not need to accept the point that alcohol is a drug in order to adopt low-risk choices. If people do not need to accept the point in order to make low-risk choices, and if discussing the point becomes a barrier to some people moving with us to accept low-risk choices, then the point is best left out of a prevention program. We must distinguish between what we want people to know and what needs to be presented to meet them where they are so that we can help them move to where they need to go with the least possible disruption.

CONCLUSION

Maximizing behavior change requires careful attention to the process of planned change and to persuasion principles. The majority of time and effort should be in the unfreezing and refreezing stages of change. Successful prevention programs and activities focus on a clear understanding of behavioral objectives and a careful analysis of the barriers to adopting behavioral goals. Thus, prevention activities should target a specific audience with a specific message. Prevention that focuses on simply changing what people know about alcohol and drugs will miss an opportunity to change what people actually do.

Special Issues in Lifestyle Risk Reduction

An ounce of prevention is worth a pound of cure.

—Anonymous

Any innovative prevention model predictably raises concerns and questions about how the model applies to particular situations, substances, or groups. In this chapter, we provide an overview of six special issues that often arise in implementing the Lifestyle Risk Reduction Model. People who have been working from a zero-tolerance perspective for youth have understandable questions about teaching lifetime low-risk guidelines to people under age 21. They also may wonder how Lifestyle Risk Reduction differs from "responsible drinking" and "harm reduction" approaches. Others have questions about how Lifestyle Risk Reduction addresses illicit drugs and the challenges of cultural diversity. This chapter addresses these issues, as well as several others that are important for Lifestyle Risk Reduction programs.

SPECIAL ISSUES IN TEACHING LIFETIME LOW-RISK GUIDELINES TO YOUTH

In our approach, the Five Conditions of the Lifestyle Risk Reduction Model apply to all people regardless of age. The implication is that young people will grow up learning that alcohol and drug problems occur because of the kind of choices people make, and only low-risk choices can prevent future problems. Young people need low-risk guidelines for a lifetime within the context of age-appropriate expectations. These low-risk guidelines call for abstinence from illicit drugs at all ages, using prescription drugs only under the strict supervision of a physician, and not exceeding specified quantity and frequency guidelines for alcohol. These guidelines are taught in the context of a clear expectation of abstinence for young people, and presented in a way that helps the young person understand why our society asks him or her to abstain until age 21. Most people do not have difficulty with teaching low-risk guidelines for using prescription medication, but some people object to teaching low-risk guidelines for alcohol to anyone under legal purchase age.

Certainly the zero-tolerance approach provides the simplest message for young people since it only addresses abstinence without getting into the complexities of different substances or different ages. It is also an appealing argument that anything added to the abstinence message has the potential of diluting it. However, there are several reasons for including an understanding of low-risk guidelines for a lifetime in the abstinence message. First, to prevent problems for a lifetime, not just while a person is young, prevention must address a lifetime. We cannot identify a single example of any prevention area that addresses a lifetime problem only from the perspective of childhood. An abstinence only message does not prepare young people for the reality of a world where purchasing alcohol is socially acceptable and legal after age 21. If they are raised with an abstinence only message, they are not likely to return to parents, teachers or prevention workers at age 21 and ask for information that was not taught when they were under legal purchase age. As discussed in Chapter 1, failing to prepare young people for a society where alcohol is available and legal has contributed to the dichotomizing of drinking in college into abstaining and heavy drinking.

In addition, approaches that withhold lifelong, lifesaving information from young people have missed an opportunity to make the information universally known to adults, since there is no "system" in the United States that reaches all adults beyond school age. There is no mechanism for making a message widely known to adults without also making it known to youth. The era of "adult secrets" that protect children from the "ugly side" of life is gone. Children grow up today exposed to the same things adults are and we cannot shield them. If we don't prepare them to make sense of the choices they will face, they will face the future unprepared.

We also face the reality that not all young people accept the message of abstinence until age 21. Teaching low-risk guidelines is an essential part of reducing high-risk use among these youth. This is supported by the fact that even after more than a decade of zero-tolerance prevention, a majority of American youth choose to use alcohol before age 21. We also know that the age range with the greatest percentage of high-risk drinking, and highest rate of alcohol-related problems, begins at age 18, in spite of a national purchase age of 21. There is also evidence that prevention only addressing abstinence is succeeding primarily in convincing the lightest drinkers to abstain, while the heaviest drinkers are drinking more.

For a majority of states, while the purchase of alcohol is illegal until age 21, consumption is not illegal in all cases. Many states have laws that allow parents to serve alcohol to minor children in their home; in some states, drinking in public places is not illegal if the parent is serving the alcohol. In fact, parents from some cultures have done this for centuries. They are not violating the law, their values, their religion, or their traditions. Further, if parents make low-risk drinking choices, there is no evidence that small amounts of alcohol increases the child's risk of experiencing problems with alcohol in later life. In fact, some evidence shows that such teens may actually drink less and have lower rates of problems. Zero-tolerance prevention strategies are often prefaced with the statement, "Since it is illegal for those under age 21 to drink . . . ," but this is not universal, even in the United States.

The objection to teaching low-risk guidelines to those under 21 is based on the fear that teaching anything other than abstinence will send a mixed message and increase alcohol use by young people.[1] The most direct way to check the accuracy of this fear is to examine prevention efforts in this country that utilize a Lifestyle Risk Reduction approach and have taught low-risk guidelines to those under age 21. Since the zero-tolerance approach has predominated, only a few programs have been evaluated. To our knowledge, the only evaluations available have been carried out on programs developed by Prevention Research Institute (Daugherty & O'Bryan, 1986). To date, none of these evaluations have been published in peer-reviewed journals, and several have important limitations including high drop out/attrition, short-term follow-ups, and lack of randomization. Taken as a whole, these evaluations indicate that the approach succeeds in altering attitudes, increasing abstinence, and reducing high-risk drinking in a variety of audiences (Thompson, 1996).

Another indicator of the success of this approach comes from international data and experience. Few cultures formally teach low-risk guidelines for alcohol, but numerous cultures allow teens to drink and informal norms evolve to guide that consumption. We find no evidence that youth consumption and problems are any higher in those cultures than in our own, and they may actually be lower. This does not imply that our culture should encourage youth to drink. We made that mistake during the "responsible drinking" prevention era and discovered that one culture's drinking practices cannot simply be introduced to our own. We do not have the full set of norms, cultural beliefs, and sanctions to support those practices. However, the experiences of other cultures suggest that there is no inherent danger in young people having information about low-risk guidelines.

Taken as a whole, there are compelling reasons to support the belief that young people should grow up learning risk reduction information, including lifetime low-risk guidelines and clear expectations for their behavior as young people. It is important to deliver this information in a way that helps young people understand and accept the different expectations that our culture holds for people at different ages.

[1]Others may object on the basis that it is not consistent with federal guidelines that call for a zero-tolerance message for youth. We agree that "no use" by adolescents should be a primary message, but within a Lifestyle Risk Reduction approach. Zero tolerance does not address the lifespan.

HOW DOES LIFESTYLE RISK REDUCTION DIFFER FROM RESPONSIBLE DRINKING?

Teaching lifetime low-risk guidelines for alcohol, especially to youth, raises questions for some people about whether or not Lifestyle Risk Reduction is just another way to teach responsible drinking. The approaches are very different, and it is important to make the distinction between the two since, for good reasons, responsible drinking education has been targeted for elimination by proponents of youth-focused prevention.

Responsible drinking education has a complex history. This education represented a specific model, the Normative/Socio-Cultural Model, with its own articulations of cause and prevention strategies. Most people who oppose responsible drinking are unaware of this history and the fact that "responsible drinking" is not just a phrase. We find few people who know what the model is and why it failed. Instead, the tendency is to interpret responsible drinking to simply be that amorphous area between abstinence and problems. Since people "know" that responsible drinking education was harmful, they assume that all prevention efforts that are not "abstinence only" must be responsible drinking and, for reasons unknown, such approaches are "bad."

The version of the Normative Model that incorporated responsible drinking education was based on cross-cultural research. This research (Plaut, 1967), conducted primarily from 1940 to 1960, found that cultures with low rates of alcoholism integrated alcohol into everyday life with clear norms and expectations for use. Children were introduced to alcohol at home at a young age. Drinking was an unemotional topic and a normal part of religious observance, meals, and celebrations, but drunkenness was generally unacceptable. On the other hand, cultures with higher rates of alcohol problems were more conflicted about drinking and people were introduced to alcohol outside the home, typically at an older age. Norms regarding the use of alcohol were not clear. Based on these findings, responsible drinking programs attempted to integrate alcohol as a normal part of society. The methods were based on the assumption that social context was more important than quantity and frequency in determining risk for problems related to drinking. Why people drank, when they drank, and drinking circumstances were deemed more important than how much and how often a person drank. In addition, no one could tell anyone else what was responsible drinking for them. Each person identified what was responsible using the general guideline of "any drinking that did not lead to problems." Immediate outcomes of drinking were used as a practical measure of "how much is too much drinking," which led to impairment problems as the prevention focus, largely ignoring possible long-term health problems. It was implicit that parents, churches, and schools could only teach young people to be responsible and then give them freedom to decide. Responsible drinking also suggested that while it is vital for a society to develop drinking norms, society cannot dictate the norms. Neither could abstainers develop the norms. Responsible drinking theory suggested that norms must come from those who drink, and would evolve through discussion designed to help individuals and small groups develop their own definition of responsible drinking. If drinkers developed the norms themselves, they were more likely to follow them.

If this sounds like a "do your own thing" approach to prevention, keep in mind that responsible drinking education evolved in the 1960s and reflected the time in which it was first developed. In practice, responsible drinking prevention led to young people from junior high to college being told such things as, "Making responsible choices and responsible decisions is something that each individual must do for him- or herself. No one can tell you what responsible behavior is for you" (Engs, 1987). Consistent with this philosophy, one popular responsible drinking curriculum (Mills, Deutsch, & DiCicco, 1978) instructed fourth-graders to discuss what would be "moderate drinking" and come to their own conclusions. They were directed to discuss why two drinks might be moderate for adults or teens, but not for younger children. Fifth-graders were asked to determine what rules they would make for themselves about drinking, and sixth-graders were asked to brainstorm a list of reasons why 11-year olds might drink, and to divide the list into reasons that were okay and not okay. Sixth-graders were also asked to role-play a wedding in which the child who is "almost 12" wanted to have a "good time" and have a couple of drinks. The role-play instructed, "You know you won't overdo it. You behave like an adult in a lot of other ways; your parents should trust you to drink responsibly, too." The students were left to take the role-play in whatever direction they wanted. Seventh-graders were asked to role-play two 15-year-olds asking someone older to buy alcohol so they could celebrate a birthday. The students playing the 15-year-olds were asked, "What do you do? How do you go about asking him if he'll buy for you?" The seventh grader role-playing the "22-year-old married man" who was being asked to buy was instructed that the students look to be age 16. The curriculum asks him to consider questions such as, "Did you drink at age 16? Would you buy for them if they asked you?" Again, the students were left to take the role-play in any direction. No guidance was given on the desired outcome.

Proponents of zero-tolerance prevention assume that responsible drinking education failed because it addressed drinking rather than abstaining. We suggest that responsible drinking education failed, not because it addressed the reality that people drink, but because it addressed that reality in a way that encouraged drinking as well as high-risk consumption.

In important ways, Lifestyle Risk Reduction is the opposite of responsible drinking education. Lifestyle Risk Reduction teaches that when, why, and under what circumstances a person drinks is not as important as the quantity and frequency of drinking. Lifestyle Risk Reduction teaches that abstinence is one of the low-risk quantity and frequency choices. Instead of waiting for a problem to develop to know that a choice is "irresponsible," Lifestyle Risk Reduction teaches people how to avoid the risk of a problem. Lifestyle Risk Reduction also emphasizes that research determines what is low risk, and that informed prevention can help people of all ages understand age-appropriate low-risk choices, taught within the context of the law, family values, and religious beliefs. Parents, churches and schools are supported in having both the right and the responsibility to teach risk reduction information with clear expectations for age-appropriate low-risk choices. In short, while a person may make the value judgment that Lifestyle Risk Reduction is "responsible," it bears no similarity to the Responsible Drinking approach.

HOW DOES LIFESTYLE RISK REDUCTION DIFFER FROM HARM REDUCTION?

Harm Reduction, a more recent development in prevention, is sometimes confused with Lifestyle Risk Reduction. The confusion increases as more advocates of Harm Reduction refer to it as Risk Reduction (Duncan, Nicholson, Patrick, Hawkins, & Petosa, 1994). The difference is simple. As stated by Marlatt, Somers, and Tapert (1993), harm reduction is, "The application of methods designed to reduce the harm (and risk of harm) associated with ongoing or active addictive behaviors." In other words, harm reduction does not focus on reducing high-risk alcohol or drug use, it focuses on keeping use from causing problems. An example might be needle exchange programs for intravenous drug users. These programs do nothing to reduce the use of drugs but may prevent AIDS, hepatitis, and other needle-borne infections. Another example is the promotion of designated driver programs that do not attempt to reduce drinking, but may reduce drunk driving arrests and motor vehicle crashes.

Lifestyle Risk Reduction, on the other hand, targets reducing high-risk drug use itself. More accurately, it focuses on simultaneously increasing the rate of abstinence, delaying the age of onset of use, and reducing high-risk use.

RISK REDUCTION AND ILLEGAL DRUGS

The need for Lifestyle Risk Reduction is most clearly evident, and most easily illustrated, for alcohol. It is not always immediately clear to people how the Lifestyle Risk Reduction Model applies to illegal drugs. Aside from the issue of legality, there are several reasons that the only low-risk guideline given for illicit drugs is abstinence. First, there are realistic limitations that make it very difficult to identify low-risk quantities of any illegal substance. Alcohol content in various alcoholic beverages is relatively standardized and there are millions of people worldwide who drink some alcohol with some degree of regularity and do not use any illegal drugs. It is, therefore, possible to find large enough populations to study to determine the long-term risk associated with specific patterns of drinking. For illicit drug use, this is more difficult. People who use illegal drugs tend to use multiple substances over time which makes outcomes of use difficult to study.

Low-risk guidelines for use of alcohol are designed to address both health and impairment problems. By definition, then, any amount of alcohol that increases risk for health problems or results in impairment is high risk. In part, it is possible to determine, and meaningful to provide, low-risk guidelines for alcohol because many people find it desirable to drink small amounts of alcohol without becoming intoxicated. Think back to the data on alcohol consumption presented in Chapter 2. Thirty percent of the drinkers consume 90 percent of the alcohol. This 30 percent is typically drinking high-risk quantities whenever they drink. Their primary motive for drinking is to alter their consciousness. However, 70 percent of the drinkers only consume 10 percent of the alcohol. The majority of these people are drinking low-risk quantities when they drink. They are not impaired nor are they endangering their health. Most of them are using alcohol for some purpose other than altering consciousness. They may have a glass of wine with dinner or a beer after mowing the yard. On the other hand, the primary purpose of using most illegal drugs is to alter consciousness. By definition, whenever consciousness is altered, impairment is present. Thus, for most illegal drugs, any amount that people generally find desirable to use causes impairment and is high risk. It might be theoretically possible to identify quantities of cocaine, for example, that are low-risk for health and impairment. However, it would be such a small amount that it would not provide the high that people seek. There would be little motivation to use. For very practical reasons, then, the only low-risk guideline for illegal drugs is abstinence.

The fact that there is no low-risk use of illicit drugs does not change the need for adopting a goal of reducing high-risk use. This has been implicitly recognized in the establishment of national goals for drug abuse as listed in the National Drug Control Strategy (1996). Multiple goals refer to reducing levels of illegal drug abuse. This is synonymous with reducing high-risk drug use, which is important not only to reduce use-related problems, but also to minimize escalation of use.

However, the differences in alcohol and illegal drugs do not stop with definitions. It has been theorized for some time that the social acceptability of a substance will, to a large extent, determine the psychosocial profile of the user: the more normative the substance, the more normative the profile of the "typical" user. When using a substance is normative, both abstainers and heavy users are likely to exhibit a nonnormative psychosocial profile, while light users are more likely to have a normative profile. On the other hand, the less socially acceptable a substance, the less normative the psychosocial profile of both light and heavy users will be and the more normative the profile of nonusers. Significant data support these observations (Cahalan & Room, 1974; Newcomb & Bentler, 1988). Of practical interest, the "typical" illicit drug user tends to be more antisocial, more hostile, and more rebellious than the "typical" drinker.[2]

Prevention theory in the last two decades has generally focused on the similarities in users and in substances. Using the logic that all abused substances are similar, and encouraged by the reality that many people abuse both alcohol and drugs, prevention has been designed to address all substances simultaneously. Yet, as noted earlier, the prevention impact has not been uniform across substances or ages, which suggests that one approach may not fit the needs of all substances, all people, and all ages. Instead of focusing on the similarities between users and substances, it seems logical to also focus on the differences, and to develop prevention strategies that reflect both.

Looking at the general population, the "typical" person who only drinks alcohol, the "typical" person who uses crack, the "typical" person who uses only marijuana, and the "typical" person who

[2]It is widely believed that the "typical drinker" no longer exists among young drinkers and has been replaced by the "multiple substance user." However, one only needs to compare the percent who drink alcohol and the percent who use illegal drugs to see that there are still many people who only drink alcohol, or who only use illicit drugs on rare occasions. It is also widely believed that young people do not drink low-risk quantities—when they drink they drink to get drunk. Again, the data do not support the perception. A larger percentage of young people do drink to get drunk and "binge" drink, compared with adults. However, the majority of young people do not do so, and a large percentage of those who sometimes binge, do so only on occasion.

uses heroin do not usually have the same psychosocial profile. There are reasons why some people prefer sedatives, while others prefer stimulants or hallucinogens. We need to learn more about the similarities and differences between different categories of drug users to design meaningful prevention for each.

The Social Influences Model and the Personal and Social Skills Model have shown results for reducing tobacco, alcohol, and marijuana use among young children and early teens. Based on preliminary data and anecdotal information, the Lifestyle Risk Reduction Model appears to have meaningful results for alcohol with teens, young adults, and adults. The success to date has come largely from understanding similarities between substances and users. We believe future success will come largely from better understanding the differences between substances and users.

LIFESTYLE RISK REDUCTION AND CULTURAL DIVERSITY

The differences that we have just discussed are for groups of drug users where variation exists for the type of drug being used. Cultural diversity occurs within a population using the same substance. These differences may be related to racial, ethnic, religious, geographic, religious or other factors. How would these differences be taken into account when using a Lifestyle Risk Reduction approach?

The Lifestyle Risk Reduction Model focuses on what is the same for all people and what is likely to be different. The central tenets of the model appear to be universal. The formula, "biology + quantity and frequency = risk" applies to everyone. The five conditions—(1) it could happen to me, my choices matter; (2) I know what to do; (3) people around me support low-risk choices; (4) I want to make low-risk choices; and (5) I have the skills I need—are also a universal necessity for risk reduction. The way in which they are applied for any particular group may vary, with the greatest difference being in Conditions Three, Four, and Five. While different language, analogies, and examples are needed for different populations, there is no need for changes in the Lifestyle Risk Reduction approach to fulfill Conditions One and Two: it could happen to me, my choices matter, and I know what to do. On the other hand, a cultural environment that supports either low-risk or high-risk choices, and the personal traits that must be appealed to and strengthened, can vary significantly to affect Conditions Three, Four, and Five. For example, we have observed a much greater difference in the degree to which Hispanic males view drinking as a sign of personal strength, and how this view is often supported and protected by Hispanic females. Therefore, in our experience, it is not unusual for Hispanic females to respond to the low-risk guidelines by saying, "This is fine for me, but not my husband. I could never expect him to do this." This presents greater challenges in establishing Condition Three—social support—for Hispanic males. On the other hand, there appears to be greater support for abstinence among African-American women. In our experience, this translates more easily into social support for low-risk choices by African-American males and provides a basis for strengthening Condition Three among African-American males. Thus, our experience indicates that there are very different social influences to work with in these two cultures. We have also found that affluent communities present challenges for teen alcohol use. On one hand, it is easier to mobilize parent involvement. On the other hand, these communities are often very social for both adults and teens. They may have formal parties with young children in attendance. Youth in these communities often have a considerable amount of spending money and unsupervised time. Unlike communities characterized by less affluence, many of the forces that encourage drinking and drug use among teens in affluent communities are looked on as positive, and parents are hesitant to change them.

Abstaining religious groups present another interesting prevention opportunity. As a group members have a very high rate of abstaining; however, there is a higher than expected rate of problems among their members who do drink, especially if they are not actively involved in the religious group. Because of the abstinence stance, members of the group may initially be opposed to teaching low-risk guidelines. Helping them see this need involves a different approach to accomplishing Condition One—it could happen to me. The belief is that, "It can't happen to us because we don't drink."

Once they understand that a significant percentage do drink, and that those who drink may experience a higher rate of problems, it becomes easier for them to accept the need for risk reduction. In our experience, it has been especially useful to share research showing that young people from abstaining religious groups who are not actively involved tend to drink more. Parents know that their own children may go through a time of rejecting their religious upbringing, and they want to protect their children during this time. Risk reduction prevention can help accomplish this, but it must be presented within a context that supports the abstinence position of the church.

LIFESTYLE RISK REDUCTION AND THE TWO PREVENTION QUESTIONS

We have already noted that the Lifestyle Risk Reduction formula addresses both use and problems. The basic formula, "biology + quantity and frequency," answers the question, "What causes problems?" The psychological and social influence arrows answer the question, "What causes use?" (see Fig. 3.2). We would now like to expand on how the model addresses these questions.

Once use occurs, there are certain biological factors that can also influence quantity/frequency choices (see Fig. 7.1). For example, biological factors will cause differences in response to alcohol causing some people to become ill, such as the flushing response that is common among people of Asian decent (Akutsu, Sue, Zane, & Nakamura, 1989). This very negative biological response makes drinking so unpleasant that it is protective against alcoholism (Crabb, Edenberg, Thomasson, & Li, 1995). Few people who have a severe flushing response develop alcoholism. Other people have a biological response on the other end of the pleasure continuum which causes them to have an unusually pleasant response to alcohol. There is evidence that children of alcoholics tend to rate their first drinking experiences as being more pleasurable than do children of nonalcoholics. There is also evidence that children of alcoholics tend to experience greater relaxation, experience less impairment, are less aware of impairment when it

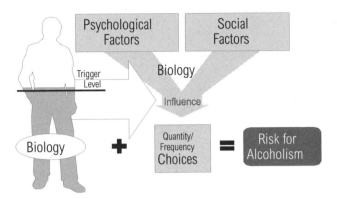

Figure 7.1.   Once use occurs, biology becomes an important influence.

does occur, and develop tolerance more rapidly (Sher, 1994). It is understandable that these experiences would influence higher levels of consumption.

Taste is another example of a biological influence on drinking choices. Those who do not like the taste of beer often find it hard to imagine that other people prefer the taste of beer to a soft drink. If no one liked the taste of beer, there would likely be no market for alcohol-free beer.

Tolerance is another example. If people are drinking for a particular effect, their tolerance levels will govern how much alcohol it takes to achieve the sought after effect.

But the initial decision to drink, and much of our later drinking behavior, is primarily influenced by psychosocial factors, as described earlier. It is appropriate, then, that most prevention efforts have focused on psychosocial influences. However, the Lifestyle Risk Reduction Model suggests that it is important to tie those efforts to an understanding of what is low risk and an understanding of how problems develop. Only biology and quantity/frequency choices have a direct impact on developing the health problem. Psychological and social influences play an indirect role. As such, they are like the mythical multiheaded Hydra: One or two heads can be cut off, yet there are still four or five heads left to "bite."

The history of psychosocial approaches to prevention is filled with examples of prevention programs that successfully changed attitudes, knowledge, decision-making ability, self-esteem, communication skills or other theoretically important psychosocial measures, but made no impact on drinking or drug-taking behavior (Ellickson & Robyn, 1987; Falck & Craig, 1988; Hansen et al., 1988). For example, a person may have strong family support, attend church regularly, have great coping skills and a healthy self-concept, but if he believes that risk for alcoholism is due to the kind of person he is, and does not understand the risk in consuming six drinks a day, then he is headed for trouble.

The most important psychosocial factors are those that most directly influence use. These include attitudes and beliefs about the substance and its use. We believe that prevention activities must focus directly on instilling an understanding of the basic part of the formula, Biology + Quantity/Frequency, if they are to succeed.

Prevention efforts have suffered from what might be thought of as "over-pathologizing" the risk for problems. The belief has been that alcohol and drug problems are the result of pathology, poverty, chaotic family life, and/or poor coping skills. There is little doubt that all these factors can play a role, but so can affluence, celebrations, and drinking for fun. Accurate drinking histories reveal that many people who develop alcoholism initially drink primarily because it is pleasurable. Drinking to cope with problems does not occur until well into the progression of the alcoholism. Prevention, then, must also focus on the pleasurable part of the experience as well as the pathology. People engage in high-risk drinking for many different reasons. If we try to change the behavior indirectly by focusing only on the psychosocial reasons for use, it is likely that we can have success in changing the influences without changing enough of them to change the behavior.

SUMMARY

There are special issues to consider with any prevention model. When applying the Lifestyle Risk Reduction Model for those under age 21, lifetime guidelines are taught within the context of age-appropriate expectations. Applying the model to illegal drugs and to special populations requires attention to the similarities and differences in substances and in groups. Evaluating Life-style Risk Reduction programs incorporates attention to the three behavioral goals and the related attitudes.

8

Concluding Remarks

This book was written for practitioners, program developers, and students who are interested in preventing alcohol and drug problems. The information focuses on a prevention intervention which can be used to decrease the high-risk use of substances across the lifespan. Selected popular prevention approaches for youth and associated research are reviewed. The integrating model approach which is presented, called Lifestyle Risk Reduction, provides tangible ways to assist individuals in altering their high-risk behaviors, with the goal of reducing their risk for alcohol and drug problems across the lifespan.

Preventing alcohol and drug problems can be straightforward when the focus is on youth prevention and education, which is the current approach in the United States. However, alcohol and drug prevention is more complicated when the focus is expanded to all ages. Simplicity from one point of view, with the focus on youth, provides an opportunity for a quick fix and an easy solution. However, we believe that the youth-focused prevention approach should be complemented with a lifespan approach to prevent alcohol and drug problems as individuals develop and change in their lifespans. In our opinion, prevention information and interventions should also be specific and applicable for a variety of individuals.

Little has been written about prevention with adults, and limited information is available about lifespan prevention, which is a new and different approach to prevention for many people. In fact, when most people think about alcohol and drug prevention, they think about kids and young people. The lifespan approach targets kids and youth as well as young adults and adults. It is a way of thinking about problems associated with use which underscores the important message of no use for underage persons, and no use of illegal drugs for anyone. In our experience, thinking about prevention that focuses only on one part of the lifespan can produce mixed messages and inconsistencies. For example, responsible use messages in the United States originated from adult-focused research and prevention theory in the 1970s. When responsible use messages were interpreted for kids and youth, the results were very negative. How could we teach young people to make responsible decisions about alcohol and drug use when they are not legally able to use alcohol? What about responsible use of illegal drugs? One of the results from a responsible use message in the United States was a zero-tolerance approach to prevention that focused almost exclusively on youth, and created practical and conceptual problems for prevention with adults and young adults.

Prevention involves individual choices and therefore is further complicated as we examine the need to take a hard look at personal attitudes and behaviors about preventing alcohol and drug problems. In the past decade, there has been an emphasis on health promotion and disease prevention in the United States. That emphasis incorporates a more holistic approach for prevention within a context of individual behavioral changes. Preventing heart disease is the example frequently used, and the one we used. Although oversimplified, there are believers and nonbelievers in prevention. On one hand, a believer in prevention is the kind of person who watches his or her diet to control heart disease, exercises, wears a seat belt automatically, and is aware of personal safety. This person is more receptive to prevention messages and can be persuaded more easily to incorporate quantity and frequency choice information as a part of his or her lifestyle. A nonbeliever in prevention, on the other hand, can be described as a risk-taker who approaches life in a swashbuckling way. In fact, nonbelievers may defy prevention recommendations and, as adults, maintain the attitude they had as adolescents—that they are invincible. Prevention messages are more difficult for nonbelievers to hear and act on, especially youth.

MAJOR POINTS OF EMPHASIS

The following bullets provide a quick reference for the major points made in this volume:

- Youth are not getting prevention messages that can last throughout their lifespans.
- Youth-focused prevention should be complemented with lifespan prevention.
- Alcohol and drug prevention should focus on problems related to alcohol and drugs.
- Legitimate differences exist in prevention for alcohol and prevention for illegal drugs.
- There is a gap in prevention because high-risk use is not being addressed.
- Responsible use of alcohol or drugs is not a viable prevention approach.
- Changing behaviors related to alcohol and drug use can be very complex.
- Persuasion plays an important role in prevention.
- Research should be used both to develop and evaluate prevention interventions.
- People must keep quantity and frequency choices clearly in their minds when they drink alcohol, considering their biological triggers in addition to psychological and social factors.
- Responsible use of substances is not part of the Lifestyle Risk Reduction approach and the emphasis is not on harm reduction.

HELPFUL HINTS FOR THE PRACTITIONER AND OTHERS

So what can we do to help individuals focus on their high-risk choices related to alcohol use or illegal drug use? The choice is clearly theirs, but their choice to engage in high-risk behavior is something that many of us believe must be addressed directly.

A key is, of course, recognition and understanding that preventing problems related to alcohol and illegal drugs is personal. The first phase in the change process is described as unfreezing current attitudes and values. Unfreezing takes time and is important. It should be noted that it may not be possible to accomplish this unfreezing task quickly, and it may take more time than a practitioner may be able to invest. From the Lifestyle Risk Reduction point of view, it is important for the person to know that their high-risk choices are related to *quantity choices* and *frequency choices*. These choices determine their risk reinforcement, especially when an individual's biology is discussed as the trigger level and psychological factors and social factors are personalized and incorporated.

An important first step in this process, as presented in Figure 3.2, is talking about a recognition of the biological risk role that heredity/genetics play in decisions related to drinking choices and the process of making high-risk drinking choices. For example, are parents, grandparents, or members of the individual's immediate family alcohol dependent? Do they use illegal drugs? Do they believe they can "hold their liquor"? In our opinion each of us should know our biological trigger level for risk. However, we need to know more than just that to make good decisions about alcohol. Psychological and social factors related to use are also important, and they vary for each of us. These are personal factors related to why a person drinks and in what situations a person drinks.

With limited time available, overviewing the risk reduction approach presented in Figure 6.1 may be all that is possible. However, it is recommended that more time be used to give a complete "dose" of the intervention. With additional time, further discussion and reinforcement of the importance of choice situations is possible. This should take into account the person's biological trigger level, psychological factors, and social factors within high-risk quantity and frequency choices. However, the point is clear. The door must be opened, information should be provided that is clear and non-judgmental, and it should be personalized to pinpoint clearly the individual's risk for alcohol and other drug problems.

References

Akutsu, P. D., Sue, S., Zane, N. W. S., & Nakamura, C. Y. (1989). Ethnic differences in alcohol consumption among Asians and Caucasians in the United States: An investigation of cultural and physiological factors. *Journal of Studies on Alcohol, 50,* 261–267.

Allen, D. N., Sprenkel, D. G., & Vitale, P. A. (1994). Reactance theory and alcohol consumption laws: Further confirmation among collegiate alcohol consumers. *Journal of Studies on Alcohol, 55,* 34–40.

American Psychiatric Association. (1987). *Diagnostic and statistical manual of mental disorders: DSM-III-R.* Washington, DC: Author.

Anthony, J. C., & Helzer, J. E. (1991). Syndromes of drug abuse and dependence. In L. N. Robins & D. A. Regier (eds.), *Psychiatric disorders in America* (pp. 116–154), New York: The Free Press.

Bachman, J., Johnston, L., & O'Malley, P. (1988). Explaining the recent decline in marijuana use: Differentiating the effects of perceived risks, disapproval, and general lifestyle factors. *Journal of Health and Social Behavior, 29,* 92–112.

Bales, R. F. (1944). *The "fixation factor" in alcohol addiction: An hypothesis derived from a comparative study of Irish and Jewish social norms.* New York: Arno Press.

Barnes, G. E. (1979). The alcoholic personality: A reanalysis of the literature. *Journal of Studies on Alcohol, 40,* 571–634.

Begleiter, H., & Kissin, B. (eds.). (1996). *The Pharmacology of Alcohol and Alcohol Dependence.* New York: Oxford University Press.

Berman, S.M., Whipple, S. M., Fitch, R. I., & Noble, E. P. (1993). P3 in young boys as a predictor of adolescent substance use. *Alcohol 10,* 69–76.

Bernard, B. (1994). Guides for the journey from risk to resilience. *Western Center News, 7. Portland, OR: Western Regional Center Drug-Free Schools and Communities, Northwest Regional Educational Laboratory.*

Berrueta-Clement, J. R., Schweinhart, L. J., Barness, W. S. M., & Weikart, D. P. (1983). *The effects of early education intervention on crime and delinquency in adolescence and early adulthood.* Ypsilanti, MI: Center for the Study of Public Policies for Young Children.

Botvin, G. J. (1990). Substance abuse prevention: Theory, practice, and effectiveness. In M. Tonry & J. Q. Wilson (Eds.), *Drugs and crime* (pp. 461–519), Chicago: The University of Chicago Press.

163

Brochu, S., & Souliere, M. (1988). Long-term evaluation of a life skills approach for alcohol and drug abuse prevention. *Journal of Drug Education, 18,* 311–331.

Brown, J. H., D'Emidio-Caston, M., & Pollard, J. A. (1997). Students and substances: Social power in drug education. *Educational Evaluation and Policy Analysis, 19,* 65–82.

Burkett, S. (1977). Parental influence and adolescent alcohol and marijuana use. *Journal of Drug Issues, 7,* 263–273.

Cadoret, R. J., & Gath, A. (1978). Inheritance of alcoholism in adoptees. *British Journal Psychiatry, 132,* 252–258.

Cahalan, D., & Room, R. (1974). Problem drinking among American men. *Monograph No. 7 Rutgers Center for Alcohol Studies.* New Haven: College and University Press.

Carr, C. N., Kennedy, S. R., & Dimick, K. M. (1996). Alcohol usage among high school athletes. *The Prevention Researcher, 3,* 3–6.

Carver, U. C. (1982). Alcohol attitudes of low-risk and high-risk drunken behavior of high-school seniors. Ph.D. diss., University of Alabama.

Center for Substance Abuse Prevention. (1997). *Secretary's youth substance abuse prevention initiative, resource papers.* Regional Technical Assistance Workshop Pre-Publication Documents, Substance Abuse and Mental Health Services Administration. Washington, DC: U.S. Department of Health and Human Services.

Chassin, L., Rogosch, F., Barrera, M. (1991). Substance use and symptomatology among adolescent children of alcoholics. *Journal of Abnormal Psychology, 100,* 449–463.

Cherpitel, C. J. (1993). Alcohol, injury, and risk-taking behavior: Data from a national sample. *Alcoholism: Clinical and Experimental Research, 17,* 762–766.

Cisin, I., & Cahalan, D. (1968). Comparison of abstainers and heavy drinkers. In J. Cole (ed.), *Clinical research in alcoholism: Psychiatric research reports of the American Psychiatric Association* (pp. 10–21). Washington, DC: American Psychiatric Association.

Clark, F. A. (1992). *Great American Bathroom Book. Compact classics, Volume I.* Salt Lake City, Utah.

Clark, W. B., & Hilton, M. E. (Eds.). (1991). *Alcohol in America: Drinking practices and problems.* Albany, NY: SUNY Press.

Clayton, R. R. (1984). Multiple drug use: Epidemiology, correlates, and consequences. In M. Galanter (Ed.), *Recent developments in alcoholism, 4* (pp. 7–38). New York: Plenum Press.

Clayton, R. R., Cattarello, A., Day, E., & Walden, K. (1991). Sensation seeking as a potential mediating variable for school-based prevention intervention: A two-year follow-up of DARE. *Health Communication, 3,* 229–239.

Cloninger, R., Bohman, M., & Sigvardsson, S. (1981). Inheritance of alcohol abuse. *Archives of General Psychiatry, 38,* 861–868.

Cloninger, C. R., Sigvardsson, S., & Bohman, M. (1988). Childhood personality predicts alcohol abuse in young adults. *Alcoholism: Clinical and Experimental Research, 12,* 494–505.

Crabb, D. W., Edenberg, H. J., Thomasson, H. R., & Li, T. K. (1995). Genetic factors that reduce risk for developing alcoholism in animals and humans. In H. Begleiter & B. Kissin (Eds.), *The genetics of alcoholism* (pp. 202–220). New York: Oxford University Press.

Daugherty, R., & O'Bryan, T. (1986). *Talking about alcohol and drugs series.* Lexington, KY: Prevention Research Institute.

Daugherty, R., & O'Bryan, T. (1996). *Prime for life series.* Lexington, KY: Prevention Research Institute.

Duncan, D. F., Nicholson, T., Patrick, C., Hawkins, W., & Petosa, R. (1994). Harm reduction: An emerging new paradigm for drug education. *Journal of Drug Education, 24,* 281–290.

Dupont, R. L. (Ed.). (1989). *Stopping alcohol and other drug abuse before it starts. OSAP Prevention Monograph No. 1.* Washington, DC: U.S. Department of Health and Human Services.

Einstein, A. (1984). *Einstein: A portrait.* Corte Madera, CA: Pomegranate Artbooks.

Ellickson, P., & Robyn, A. (1987). *Toward more effective drug prevention program* (RAND note N-2666-CHF). Santa Monica, CA: The RAND Corporation.

Ellickson, P. L., & Bell, R. M. (1990). A drug prevention in junior high: A multi-site longitudinal test. *Science, 247,* 1299–1305.

Ellickson, P. L., & Hays, R. D. (1991). Antecedents of drinking among young adolescents with different alcohol use histories. *Journal of Studies on Alcohol, 52,* 398–408.

Engen, H., Richards, C., & Patterson, A. M. (1995). *An evaluation of the state of Iowa's drunk driver education curriculum: Final report.* Iowa City, IA: University of Iowa, Iowa Consortium for Substance Abuse Research and Evaluation.

Engs, R. (1987). *Alcohol and other drugs: Self-responsibility.* Bloomington: Tichenor Publishing.

Everingham, S. S., & Rydell, C. P. (1994). *Modeling the demand for cocaine* (prepared for the Office of National Drug Control Policy United States Army). Santa Monica, CA: The RAND Corporation.

Falck, R., & Craig, R. (1988). Classroom-oriented primary prevention programming for drug abuse. *Journal of Psychoactive Drugs, 20,* 403–407.

Fergusson, D. M., Lynskey, M. T., & Horwood, J. (1994). Childhood exposure to alcohol and adolescent drinking patterns. *Addiction, 89,* 1007–1016.

Fillmore, K. M., Bacon, S. D., & Hyman, M. (1979). A 27 Year Longitudinal Panel Study of Drinking by Students in College, 1949–1976; Final Report to National Institute on Alcohol Abuse and Alcoholism (Contract No. ADM 281–76–0015). Washington, DC: U. S. Government Printing Office.

Fingarette, H. (1988). *Heavy drinking: The myth of alcoholism as a disease.* Berkeley: University of California Press.

Glynn, T. J., Leukefeld, C. G., & Ludford, J. P. (Eds.). (1983). *Preventing adolescent drug abuse: Intervention strategies: A RAUS review report, DHHS publication No. ADM83-1280.* (NIDA Research Monograph No. 47). Washington, DC: U.S. Government Printing Office.

Gomberg, E. S. (1993). Gender issues. In M. Galanter (Ed.), *Recent developments in alcoholism 11* (pp. 96–107). New York: Plenum Press.

Goodwin, D. W. (1984). Studies of familial alcoholism. In D. W. Goodwin, K. T. Van Dusen, & S. A. Mednick (Eds.), *Longitudinal research in alcoholism* (pp. 97–105). Boston: Kluwer Nijhoff Publishing.

Goodwin, D. W., Schulsinger, F., Hermansen, L., Guze, S. B., & Winokur, G. (1973). Alcohol problems in adoptees raised apart from alcoholic biological parents. *Archives of General Psychiatry, 28,* 238–243.

Grant, B. F., & Dawson D. A. (1998). Age at onset of alcohol use and its association with DSM-IV alcohol abuse and dependence: Results from the National Longitudinal Alcohol Epidemiologic Survey. *Journal of Substance Abuse, 9,* 103–110.

Greenfield, T. K., Giesbrecht, N., & Kavanagh, L. (1996, May). *Drinking patterns of young adults in the US and Canada: The policy implications.* Paper presented at the 10th International Alcohol Policy Conference, Toronto, Canada.

Haines, M., & Spear, S. F. (1996). Changing the perception of the norm: A strategy to decrease binge drinking among college students. *Journal of American College Health, 45,* 134–140.

Hansen, W., Johnson, C. A., Flay, B., Graham, J., & Sobel, J. (1988). Affective and social influences approaches to the prevention of multiple substance abuse among seventh grade students. *Preventive Medicine, 17,* 135–154.

Hansen, W., Malotte, C. K., & Fielding, J. (1988). Evaluation of a tobacco and alcohol abuse prevention curriculum for adolescents. *Health Education Quarterly, 15,* 93–114.

Hansen, W. B. (1990). School-based substance abuse prevention: A review of the state of the art in curriculum, 1980–1990. Unpublished manuscript, Wake Forest University, Wake Forest, NC.

Harburg, E., DiFranceisco, W., Webster, D. W., Gleiberman, L., & Schork, A. (1990). Familial transmission of alcohol use: II. Imitation of and aversion to parent drinking (1960) by adult offspring (1977), Tecumseh, Michigan. *Journal of Studies on Alcohol, 51,* 245–256.

Hasin, D., Grant, B., Harford, T., Hilton, M., & Endicott, J. (1990). Multiple alcohol-related problems in the United States: On the rise? *Journal of Studies on Alcohol, 51,* 485–493.

Hawkins, J. D., & Catalano, R. F. (1987, March). *The Seattle Social Development Project: Progress report on a longitudinal prevention study.* Paper presented at National Institute on Drug Abuse Science Press Seminar, Seattle, Washington.

Hawkins, J. D., & Catalano, R. F. (1992). *Communities that care: Action for drug abuse prevention.* San Francisco: Jossey-Bass Publishers.

Hawkins, J. D., Lishner, D. M., & Catalano, R. F. (1985). Childhood predictors and the prevention of adolescent substance abuse. In C. L. Jones & R. F. Baattjes (Eds.), *Etiology of drug abuse: Implications for prevention* (NIDA Research Monograph No. 56, DHHS publication No. ADM85–1335, pp. 75–126). Washington DC: Government Printing Office.

Hawkins, J. D., Catalano R. F., Morrison, D. M., O'Donnell, J., Abbott, R. D., & Day, L. E. (1989, April). *The Seattle social development project: Effects of the first four years on protective factors and problem behaviors.* Paper presented at Society for Research in Child Development, Kansas City, MO.

Hesselbrock, M. N., Hesselbrock, V. M., Babor, T. F., Stabenau, J. R., Meyer, R. E., & Weidenman, M. (1984). Antisocial behavior, psychopathology and problem drinking in the natural history of alcoholism. In D. W. Goodwin, K. T. Van Dusen, & S. A. Mednick (Eds.), *Longitudinal Research in Alcoholism* (pp. 197–214). Boston: Kluwer Nijhoff Publishing.

Hill, S. E., & Steinhauer, S. (1993). Assessment of prepubertal and postpubertal boys and girls for developing alcoholism with P300 from a visual discrimination task. *Journal of Studies on Alcohol, 54,* 350–358.

Hughes, S. P., & Dodder, R. A. (1992). Changing the legal minimum drinking age: Results of a longitudinal study. *Journal of Studies on Alcohol, 53,* 568–575.

Johnson, C. A., Graham, J., Hansen, W., Flay, B., McGuigan, K., & Gee, M. (1985). *Project Smart after three years: An assessment of sixth grade and multiple year implementations.* Los Angeles, CA: University of Southern California, Institute for Health Promotion and Disease Prevention Research and Department of Preventive Medicine.

Johnson, C. A., Hansen, W., Collins, L., & Graham, J. (1986). High-school smoking prevention: Results of a three-year longitudinal study. *Journal of Behavioral Medicine, 9,* 439–452.

Johnston, L. D., O'Malley, P. M., & Bachman, J. G. (1996). *National survey results on drug use from the Monitoring the Future Study, 1975–1995.* Washington, DC: National Institute on Drug Abuse, U.S. Department of Health and Human Services.

Kaftarian, S., Kingery, P., & Mains, D. (1997). The epidemiology of youth substance abuse: Learning more by combining surveys. *Substance Abuse and Mental Health Services*

Administration Center for Substance Abuse Prevention National Prevention Network Research Conference, 10 (p. 95). Philadelphia: U.S. Government Printing Office.

Kandel, D. (1982). Epidemiological and psychosocial perspectives on adolescent drug use. *Journal of the American Academy of Child Psychiatry, 21,* 328–347.

Kilbourne, J. (Producer). (1991). *Advertising Alcohol: Calling the Shots* (2nd ed., Film). (Available from Cambridge Documentary Films, Inc., PO Box 385, Cambridge, MA 02139)

Krein, S., Overton, S., Young, M., Spreier, K., & Yolton, R. L. (1987). Effects of alcohol on event-related brain potentials produced by viewing a simulated traffic signal. *Journal American Optometric Association, 58,* 474–477.

Kubicka, L., Kozeny, J., & Zdenek, R. (1990). Alcohol abuse and its psychosocial correlates in sons of alcoholics as young men and in the general population of young men in Prague. *Journal of Studies on Alcohol, 51,* 49–58.

Levenson, M. R., Aldwin, C. M., Butcher, J. N., DeLabry, L., Workman-Daniels, K., & Bossé, R. (1990). The MAC scale in a normal population: The meaning of 'false positives'. *Journal of Studies on Alcohol, 51,* 457–462.

Lewin, K. (1947). Frontiers in group dynamics: Concept, method and reality in social science, social equilibria and social change. *Human Relations, 1,* 5–42.

Lewin, K. (1973). Force Field Analysis. In J. E. Jones & J. W. Pfeiffer (Eds.), *The 1973 annual handbook for group facilitators* (pp. 111–113). San Diego: University Associates, Inc.

LoBello, S. G., Tarpley, B. S., & Day, C. L., (1988). Credibility of sources of information about alcohol among high school students. *Journal of Alcohol and Drug Education, 33,* 68–72.

Maccoby, N., Farquhar, J. W, Wood, P. D., & Alexander, J. (1977). Reducing the risk of cardiovascular disease: Effects of a community based campaign on knowledge and behavior. *Journal of Community Health, 3,* 100–114.

Marlatt, G. A., Somers, J. M., & Tapert, S. F. (1993). Harm reduction: Application to alcohol abuse problems. *National Institute on Drug Abuse Research Monograph No. 137,* 147–166.

Marsteller, F., Falek, A., & Rolka, D. (1997). *Evaluation of Georgia DUI Risk and Recovery Program.* Atlanta, GA: Emory University, Medical School.

Martin, M. J., & Pritchard M. E. (1991). Factors associated with alcohol use in later adolescence. *Journal of Studies on Alcohol, 52,* 5–9.

McCaig, L. (1996). *Historical estimates from the drug abuse warning network: 1978–94 estimates of drug-related emergency episodes* (SAMHSA Advance Report No. 16). Rockville, MD: Substance Abuse and Mental Health Services Administration Office of Applied Studies, U.S. Department of Health and Human Services.

McCord, W., & McCord, J. (1960). *Origins of alcoholism.* Palto Alto: Stanford University Press.

McGue, M., Sharma, A., & Benson, P. (1996). Parent and sibling influences on adolescent alcohol use and misuse: Evidence from a U.S. adoption cohort. *Journal of Studies on Alcohol, 57,* 8–18.

McGuire, W. J. (1947). Communication-persuasion models for drug education. In M. Goodstadt (Ed.), *Research on methods and programs of drug education* (pp. 1–26). Toronto, Ontario: Addiction Research Foundation.

McKenna, T., & Pickens, R. (1981). Alcoholic children of alcoholics. *Journal of Studies on Alcohol, 42,* 1021–1029.

Milam, J. R., & Ketcham, K. (1981). *Under the influence: A guide to the myths and realities of alcoholism.* Seattle: Madrona Publishers, Inc.

Milgram, G. G. (1996). Responsible decision making regarding alcohol: A re-emerging prevention/education strategy for the 1990s. *Journal of Drug Education, 26,* 357–365.

Mills, D., Deutsch, C., & DiCicco, L. (1978). *Decisions about drinking: A sequential alcohol education curriculum for grades 3–12.* Somerville, MA: Caspar Alcohol Education Program in conjunction with the Somerville Public School Faculty Curriculum Team.

Murray, R. M., Clifford, C. A., & Gurling, H. M. (1983). Twin and adoption studies. In M. Galanter (Ed.), *Recent Developments in Alcoholism I* (pp. 25–48). New York: Plenum Press.

Naisbitt, John. (1982). *Megatrends.* New York: Warner Books.

The National Drug Control Strategy: The White House, Office of National Drug Control Policy, Washington, DC. 1996.

National Institute on Alcohol Abuse and Alcoholism. (1977). *Research monograph no. 3: Normative approaches to the prevention of alcohol abuse and alcoholism.* Washington, DC: U.S. Government Printing Office.

National Institute of Alcohol Abuse and Alcoholism. (1983). *Resources guide: Prevention plus: Involving schools, parents, and the community in alcohol and drug education* (DHHS Publication No. ADM83-1256). Washington, DC: U.S. Government Printing Office.

Newcomb, M. D., & Bentler, P. M. (1988). *Consequences of adolescent drug use.* Newbury Park, CA: Sage Publications.

Office of Substance Abuse Prevention. (1989). *Prevention plus II: Tools for creating and sustaining drug-free communities* (DHHS Publication No. ADM89-1649). Washington, DC: U.S. Government Printing Office.

Office of Substance Abuse Prevention. (1991). *Prevention plus III: Assessing alcohol and other drug prevention programs at the school and community level* (DHHS Publication No. ADM 91-1817). Washington, DC. U.S. Government Printing Office.

O'Hare, T. M. (1990). Drinking in college: Consumption patterns, problems, sex differences and legal drinking age. *Journal of Studies on Alcohol, 51,* 536–541.

O'Malley, P. M., & Wagenaar, A. C. (1991). Effects of minimum drinking age laws on alcohol use, related behaviors and traffic crash involvement among American youth: 1976–1987. *Journal of Studies on Alcohol, 52,* 478–491.

O'Neill, B., Williams, A., & Dubowski, K. (1983). Variability in blood alcohol concentrations: Implications for estimating individual results. *Journal of Studies on Alcohol, 44,* 222–230.

Palinkas, L. A., Atkins, C. J., Miller, C., & Ferreira, D. (1996). Social skills training for drug prevention in high-risk female adolescents. *Preventive Medicine, 25,* 692–701.

Pandina, R. J., & Johnson, V. (1990). Familial drinking history as a predictor of alcohol and drug consumption among adolescent children. *Journal of Studies on Alcohol, 50,* 245–253.

Penick, E. C., Powell, B. J., Bingham, S. F., Liskow, B. I., Miller, N. S., & Read, M.R. (1987). A comparative study of familial alcoholism. *Journal of Studies on Alcohol, 48,* 136–146.

Pentz, M. A., Dwyer, J. H., MacKinnon, D. P. , Flay, B. R., Hansen, W. B., Wang, E. Y., & Johnson, A. (1989). A multicommunity trial for primary prevention of adolescent drug abuse: Effects on drug use prevalence. *Journal of the American Medical Association, 261,* 3259–3266.

Perkins, H. W., & Berkowitz, A. D. (1986). Perceiving the community norms of alcohol use among students: Some research implications for campus alcohol education programming. *International Journal of the Addictions, 21,* 961–976.

Plaut, T. F. (1967). *Alcohol problems: A report to the nation. A report of the Cooperative Commission on Alcoholism.* New York: Oxford University Press.

Regier, D. A., Farmer, M. E., Rae, D. S., Locke, B. Z., Keith, S. J., Judd, L. L., & Goodwin, F. K. (1990). Comorbidity of mental disorders with alcohol and other drug abuse:

Results from the Epidemiologic Catchment Area (ECA) study. *Journal of the American Medical Association, 264,* 2511–2518.

Robins, L. N., & Przybeck, T. R. (1985). Age of onset of drug use as a factor in drug and other disorders. In C. L. Jones & R. F. Baattjes (Eds.), *Etiology of drug abuse: Implications for prevention* (National Institute on Drug Abuse Research Monograph No. 56, DHHS Publication No. ADM85-1335). Washington DC: U.S. Government Printing Office.

Samson, H. H., Maxwell, C. O., & Doyle, T. F. (1989). The relation of initial alcohol experiences to current alcohol consumption in a college population. *Journal of Studies on Alcohol, 50,* 254–260.

Schlegel, R. P., & Sanborn, M. D. (1979). Religious affiliation and adolescent drinking. *Journal of Studies on Alcohol, 40,* 693–703.

Schroeder, D. S , I aflin, M. T., & Wels, D. L. (1993). Is there a relationship between self-esteem and drug use? Methodological and statistical limitations of the research. *Journal of Drug Issues, 23,* 645 665.

Schuckit, M. A., & Hesselbrock, V. (1994). Alcohol dependence and anxiety disorders: What is the relationship? *American Journal of Psychiatry, 151,* 1723–1734.

Schuckit, M. A., & Smith, T. L. (1996). An 8-year follow-up of 450 sons of alcoholic and control subjects. *Archives of General Psychiatry, 53,* 202–210.

Schuckit, M.A., Goodwin, D.W., & Winokur, G. (1972). A study of alcoholism in half siblings. *American Journal Psychiatry, 128,* 122–126.

Schuckit, M. A., Irwin, M., & Brown, S. A. (1990). The history of anxiety symptoms among 171 primary alcoholics. *Journal of Studies on Alcohol, 51,* 34–41.

Schuckit, M. A., Klein, J. L., Twitchell, G. R., & Springer, L. M. (1994). Increases in alcohol-related problems for men on a college campus between 1980 and 1992. *Journal of Studies on Alcohol, 55,* 739–742.

Sehwan, K., McLeod, J. H., & Shantzis, C. (1989). An outcome evaluation of refusal skills program as a drug abuse prevention strategy. *Journal of Drug Education, 19,* 363–371.

Shain, M., Suurvali, H., & Kilty, H. L. (1980). *The parent communication project: A longitudinal study of the effects of parenting skills on children's use of alcohol final report.* Toronto, Ontario: Addiction Research Foundation.

Sher, K. J. (1994). Individual-level risk factors. In R. Zucker, G. Boyd, & J. Howard (Eds.), *The development of alcohol problems: Exploring the biopsychosocial matrix of risk* (National Institute on Drug Abuse Research Monograph No. 26, NIH Publication 94-3495, pp. 77–108). Washington, DC: U.S. Government Printing Office.

Sher, K. J., Gershuny, B. S., Peterson, L., & Raskin, G. (1997). The role of childhood stressors in the intergenerational transmission of alcohol use disorders. *Journal of Studies on Alcohol, 58,* 414–427.

Sobell, L. C., Cunningham, J. A., Sobell, M. A., & Toneatto, T. (1993). A life-span perspective on natural recovery (self-change) from alcohol problems. In J. S. Baer, G. A. Marlatt, & R. J. McMahon (Eds.), *Addictive Behaviors Across the Life Span.* Newbury Park: Sage Press, 1993.

Tarter, R. E., Hegedus, A. M., Goldstein, G., Shelly, C., & Alterman, A. I. (1984). Adolescent sons of alcoholics: Neuropsychological and personality characteristics. *Alcoholism: Clinical and Experimental Research, 8,* 216–222.

Thompson, M. L. (1996). *A review of prevention research programs: A report to the division for substance abuse, Kentucky cabinet for human resources.* Richmond, KY: Eastern Kentucky University, Department of Education.

Tobler, N. S., & Stratton, H. H. (1997). Effectiveness of school-based drug prevention programs: A meta-analysis of the research. *The Journal of Primary Prevention, 18,* 71–128.

U.S. Department of Health and Human Services. (1996). *National Household Survey on Drug Abuse: Population estimates 1995.* Rockville, MD: Substance Abuse and Mental Health Services Administration Office of Applied Studies, U.S. Department of Health and Human Services.

Vaillant, G. (1995). *The natural history of alcoholism revisited.* Cambridge, MA: Harvard University Press.

Valles, J. (1969). *From social drinking to alcoholism.* Dallas, TX: Tane Press.

Vicary, J. R. (1979). *Relating and comparing affective education and addictions prevention.* Toronto: Addiction Research Foundation.

Virkkunen, M., & Linnoila, M. (1997). Serotonin in early-onset alcoholism. In M. Galanter (Ed.), *Recent developments in alcoholism, 13* (pp. 173–189). New York: Plenum Press.

Wagenaar, A. C., & Streff, F. M. (1989). Macroeconomic conditions and alcohol-impaired driving. *Journal of Studies on Alcohol, 50,* 217–225.

Walitzer, K. S., & Sher, K. J. (1996). A prospective study of self-esteem and alcohol use disorders in early adulthood: Evidence for gender differences. *Alcoholism: Clinical and Experimental Research, 20,* 1118–1124.

Wechsler, H., & Isaac, N. (1992). 'Binge' drinkers at Massachusetts colleges. *Journal of the American Medical Association, 267,* 2929–2931.

West, L. J. (Ed.). (1984). *Alcoholism and related problems: Issues for the American public.* Englewood Cliffs, NJ: Prentice Hall.

Whipple, S. C., Parker, E. S., & Noble, E. P. (1988). An atypical neurocognitive profile in alcoholic fathers and their sons. *Journal of Studies on Alcohol, 49,* 240–244.

Index

Abstain: *see* abstinence

Abstinence, 4, 13, 15, 16, 17, 18, 20, 21, 26, 27, 31, 32, 33, 34, 35, 38, 39, 43, 44, 57, 60, 63, 65, 66, 67, 75, 85, 93, 100, 104, 105, 108, 111, 123, 126, 139, 144, 145, 146, 147, 149, 150, 151, 154, 155

Addiction, 44, 49, 50, 59, 60, 66, 70, 92, 93, 98, 101, 103, 111, 114, 134

Adoption, 53, 54, 56, 63, 64, 66, 88, 89, 90, 105, 106, 109, 123, 127

Adult independence, 40

Affective Development Model, 72

Affective education, 41, 42, 72, 73, 75, 76, 77, 84, 99, 111, 125, 131

Age 21, 2, 3, 6, 13, 26, 27, 38, 143, 144, 145, 146, 157

AIDS, 20, 99, 150

Alcohol, 2, 3, 4, 5, 6, 7, 8, 9, 10, 11, 12, 13, 14, 17, 18, 19, 21, 24, 25, 26, 27, 28, 29, 30, 31, 32, 33, 34, 35, 36, 37, 38, 39, 40, 41, 42, 43, 45, 46, 49, 50, 55, 56, 57, 58, 59, 60, 62, 66, 67, 69, 70, 72, 73, 74, 75, 77, 78, 80, 81, 82, 83, 84, 85, 86, 88, 89, 90, 91, 92, 93, 95, 96, 98, 99, 100, 101, 102, 103, 104, 105, 106, 107, 108, 110, 113, 114, 115, 119, 120, 123, 125, 126, 127, 130, 134, 135, 137, 138, 139, 141, 144, 145, 146, 147, 149, 150, 151, 152, 153, 154, 155, 156, 157, 159, 160, 161, 162

dependence, 4, 5, 9, 11, 13, 49, 50, 56, 92, 105, 110

metabolism, 103

Alcohol-related problem, 16, 18, 28, 29, 36, 57, 60, 87, 93, 99, 100, 102, 145

Alcoholism, 9, 10, 11, 24, 25, 31, 32, 36, 44, 52, 53, 54, 55, 56, 57, 58, 59, 60, 61, 62, 63, 64, 65, 66, 67, 68, 70, 83, 86, 87, 88, 89, 90, 91, 92, 93, 99, 101, 104, 105, 110, 122, 126, 129, 133, 134, 135, 140, 141, 147, 155, 157

Athlete, 25, 26, 135

Attitude, 20, 36, 61, 62, 65, 73, 76, 79, 80, 83, 84, 86, 90, 101, 109, 113, 118, 119, 121, 122, 126, 131, 137, 139, 140, 146, 157, 158, 160, 162

Bachman, 3, 19, 20, 119

Behavior change, 62, 75, 92, 106, 115, 116, 125, 131, 137, 141, 161

Bernard, 42, 83, 84

Binge, 10, 17, 30

Biological risk, 51, 52, 53, 54, 55, 56, 58, 59, 60, 68, 70, 85, 87, 92, 93, 99, 101, 102, 104, 108, 162

Bonding, 67, 80, 84, 85, 93, 100, 111

Botvin, 76, 77, 78

Changing behavior: *see* behavior change

Cigarette, 3, 70, 73, 75, 132

Clinical alcoholic personality, 59

Cloninger, 10, 54, 63, 88, 90

Cocaine, 3, 12, 17, 18, 21, 28, 29, 30, 32, 33, 37, 38, 46, 151
Cognitive dissonance, 131
College student, 14, 16, 17, 33, 62, 90, 110
Community organization, 76, 82, 109
Conduct disorder, 10, 64, 87, 88
Continuum of use, 44
Credibility, 134, 135, 136, 137
Credible source, 74, 135, 136
Cultural context, 39
Cultural diversity, 143, 153

DARE, 42, 73, 76
DATE, 34, 35
Daugherty, 8, 62, 67, 104, 126, 146
Defense, 98, 116, 121, 124, 128, 137, 138, 139, 140
Department of Education, 45
Dependence, 2, 4, 5, 9, 11, 13, 46, 49, 50, 56, 89, 92, 99, 101, 105, 110
Developmental Model, 41, 42, 67
Disease theory, 49
Distribution of Consumption Model, 96
Drinking, 3, 4, 5, 6, 7, 8, 9, 10, 13, 14, 15, 16, 17, 18, 19, 20, 21, 26, 28, 29, 30, 31, 36, 37, 38, 39, 40, 41, 42, 49, 54, 57, 58, 59, 60, 61, 62, 63, 64, 65, 66, 67, 68, 69, 70, 85, 86, 87, 89, 93, 94, 100, 104, 105, 106, 110, 111, 122, 123, 124, 126, 129, 134, 135, 136, 140, 143, 144, 145, 146, 147, 148, 149, 150, 151, 154, 155, 156, 157, 162
    behavior, 10, 13, 39, 40, 54, 57, 59, 61, 62, 64, 65, 66, 67, 85, 89, 93, 124, 148, 156, 157
    frequency, 29, 30, 57, 58, 60, 68, 69, 129, 148, 149
    high-risk, 13, 15, 16, 17, 18, 19, 20, 21, 29, 31, 36, 49, 59, 60, 61, 67, 68, 70, 86, 93, 111, 122, 123, 126, 145, 146, 149, 151, 157, 162
    parents, 58, 64, 65, 66, 67, 111, 145, 148, 154, 162
    quantity, 29, 57, 58, 60, 68, 69, 129, 148, 149
Drug-Free Schools, 20
DSM-III, 4, 56, 92
DUI, 4, 13, 103, 124
Dysfunction, 63

Early use, 4, 5, 6, 7, 8, 9, 10, 21
Elementary school, 34, 37
Engagement, 130, 131

Family, 9, 10, 11, 36, 46, 51, 53, 54, 55, 56, 58, 59, 62, 63, 66, 67, 69, 70, 73, 75, 79, 80, 83, 84, 85, 86, 87, 89, 91, 92, 93, 104, 105, 106, 108, 110, 118, 134, 138, 149, 157, 162
    disorganization, 83, 92
    environment, 53, 54
    history, 9, 10, 11, 51, 55, 56, 58, 59, 62, 79, 85, 86, 87, 91, 92, 93, 104, 134
First use, 2, 3, 6, 7, 8, 9, 10, 11, 73, 79, 88, 134
    age at, 7
    early, 6, 7, 79, 88
Five Conditions of Risk Reduction, 58
Five principles, 52, 97, 112
Flushing, 155
Force field analysis, 117, 126, 137
Formula, 51, 59, 60, 61, 68, 69, 70, 92, 93, 94, 101, 153, 155, 157
Fraternities, 90, 100
Frequency, 29, 30, 50, 51, 52, 57, 58, 59, 60, 68, 69, 70, 92, 94, 98, 99, 100, 102, 122, 129, 144, 148, 149, 153, 155, 160, 161, 162
Friend, 66, 67, 68, 69, 106, 109, 118, 135, 136

Gateway drug, 30
Gomberg, 9
Goodwin, 9, 53, 54, 58, 66, 89, 105, 134
Greenfield, 28
Group consensus, 131
Guideline, 45, 57, 58, 102, 103, 104, 105, 106, 108, 123, 143, 144, 145, 146, 147, 148, 150, 151, 154, 157

Half-sibling, 53
Hansen, 73, 75, 139, 157
Harburg, 66
Harm reduction, 143, 150, 161
Hawkins, 42, 44, 45, 66, 78, 80, 81, 85, 88, 89, 90, 91, 150
Heart disease, 24, 26, 31, 50, 51, 52, 54, 55, 56, 57, 60, 67, 70, 78, 91, 92, 96, 99, 102, 141, 160
Hesselbrock, 9, 63

High-risk, 13, 15, 16, 17, 18, 19, 20, 21, 26,
    27, 28, 29, 31, 32, 33, 34, 35, 36, 43,
    44, 46, 49, 58, 59, 60, 61, 62, 67, 68,
    69, 70, 78, 86, 92, 93, 94, 99, 100,
    101, 105, 108, 110, 111, 112, 114, 116,
    117, 118, 119, 120, 122, 123, 124,
    126, 137, 138, 139, 145, 146, 149,
    150, 151, 154, 157, 159, 161, 162
  drinking, 13, 15, 16, 17, 18, 19, 20, 21, 29,
    49, 59, 60, 61, 67, 68, 70, 86, 93, 111,
    122, 123, 126, 145, 146, 149, 151,
    157, 162
  use, 16, 18, 19, 20, 21, 26, 27, 31, 32, 33,
    34, 35, 36, 43, 44, 46, 68, 69, 92, 105,
    108, 116, 119, 124, 126, 145, 150,
    151, 159, 161

Inhalant, 2, 3, 12
Interactivity, 131
Interpersonal skill, 42, 77, 120, 125
Intervention, 25, 32, 75, 98, 110, 135, 159,
    161, 162

Johnston, 3, 12, 16, 19, 101
Just Say No, 16, 27, 32

Kandel, 4, 10

Leukefeld, 24
Lewin, 117
Lifeskills, 112
Lifestyle choice, 52, 70
Lifestyle Risk Reduction formula, 61, 68, 92,
    93, 101, 155
Low sensitivity, 56, 59
Low-risk choice, 51, 57, 60, 93, 99, 106, 108,
    109, 110, 111, 112, 114, 118, 122, 137,
    141, 144, 149, 153, 154
Low-risk guideline, 103, 105, 106, 108, 143,
    144, 145, 146, 147, 150, 151, 154

Maccoby, 31, 91
Marijuana, 3, 10, 11, 12, 19, 20, 30, 37, 38,
    46, 73, 75, 77, 85, 110, 152, 153
Marsteller, 62
McCord, 62
McGuire's persuasion process, 127, 131, 136,
    140
Memory blackout, 17

National Household Survey, 3, 17, 29, 30
Norm, 6, 8, 10, 33, 52, 65, 67, 69, 73, 74, 75,
    76, 77, 79, 80, 84, 106, 108, 119, 146,
    147, 148
Normative model, 41, 42, 147

O'Bryan, 62, 67, 104, 126, 146
Office for Substance Abuse Prevention, 45

P3 brain wave, 9, 87
Peer resistance training, 73, 74, 77, 84, 139
Peer use, 19
Perry School Project, 84
Personal and Social Skills Model, 76, 77, 81,
    113, 153
Personality, 9, 10, 11, 52, 59, 61, 63, 64, 65,
    88, 90, 118
  trait, 52, 59, 61, 65, 90, 118
Persuasion, 101, 115, 120, 121, 127, 129,
    130, 131, 132, 136, 137, 139, 140,
    141, 161
Physical damage, 101
Planned change, 141
Popular prevention model, 43
pot: see marijuana
Prevention, 1, 2, 3, 4, 5, 6, 11, 12, 13, 14, 15,
    16, 18, 19, 20, 21, 23, 24, 25, 26, 27,
    28, 29, 31, 32, 34, 35, 36, 37, 38, 39,
    40, 41, 42, 43, 44, 45, 46, 47, 49, 50,
    56, 57, 59, 60, 62, 65, 66, 67, 68, 70,
    71, 72, 78, 81, 82, 83, 84, 85, 87, 91,
    92, 93, 94, 95, 97, 98, 99, 100, 101,
    102, 104, 105, 106, 107, 108, 109,
    111, 113, 115, 116, 117, 119, 120, 121,
    122, 123, 124, 125, 126, 127, 129,
    130, 131, 132, 133, 134, 135, 136,
    137, 138, 139, 141, 143, 144, 145,
    146, 147, 148, 149, 150, 152, 153,
    154, 155, 156, 157, 159, 160, 161
  goal, 1, 11, 23, 26, 27, 32, 34, 37, 43, 107,
    108, 123, 125, 126, 131, 139, 141
  message, 23, 25, 32, 35, 36, 37, 38, 39, 45,
    46, 57, 100, 121, 122, 123, 133, 134,
    135, 137, 138, 139, 141, 144, 160, 161
  model, 41, 42, 43, 44, 46, 47, 49, 50, 65,
    67, 71, 72, 78, 81, 82, 91, 92, 93, 95,
    106, 107, 108, 113, 143, 147, 156,
    157, 159
  potential for, 28

Prevention (*cont.*)
  purpose of, 24, 25, 34, 43, 92, 115
  theory, 1, 35, 41, 43, 47, 49, 83, 91, 92, 116, 160
  zero-tolerance, 32, 38, 40, 45, 138, 145, 149, 160
Problem, 2, 4, 5, 6, 7, 8, 9, 10, 11, 13, 16, 17, 18, 19, 20, 21, 24, 25, 26, 27, 28, 29, 30, 31, 32, 34, 35, 36, 37, 38, 42, 43, 44, 45, 46, 47, 49, 50, 51, 52, 53, 55, 56, 57, 58, 59, 60, 61, 62, 64, 65, 66, 68, 69, 70, 72, 73, 79, 80, 82, 83, 85, 87, 88, 91, 92, 93, 94, 95, 96, 98, 99, 100, 101, 102, 103, 104, 105, 106, 108, 109, 112, 113, 114, 116, 119, 122, 123, 126, 135, 141, 144, 145, 146, 147, 148, 149, 150, 151, 154, 155, 156, 157, 159, 160, 161, 162
  cause, 2, 6, 21, 29, 42, 43, 44, 46, 47, 50, 57, 59, 60, 61, 65, 83, 88, 93, 101, 108, 114, 155
Prohibition Model, 41, 42
Project Alert, 42, 73, 74, 76, 112
Project Smart, 42, 73, 74, 75, 76, 112
Psychopathology, 62, 63, 64
Psychosocial factor, 44, 46, 70, 91, 94, 100, 156, 157
Public Health Model, 42, 95, 96, 97, 107

Q-sort, 126
Quantity, 29, 30, 50, 51, 52, 57, 58, 59, 60, 68, 69, 70, 92, 94, 98, 99, 100, 102, 122, 129, 144, 148, 149, 153, 155, 160, 161, 162

Recovery, 31, 49, 50, 65, 98, 104
Refreezing stage, 120, 141
Religion, 67, 145
Religious group, 65, 106, 108, 154, 155
Repetition, 75, 132, 133
Responsible use, 14, 25, 160, 161
Rhetorical question, 132
Risk and resiliency, 42, 78, 80, 81, 82, 84, 89, 91, 112
Risk factor, 5, 6, 7, 56, 78, 79, 80, 81, 82, 83, 84, 85, 86, 87, 88, 89, 90, 91, 92, 93, 94, 102
Risk for problems, 6, 28, 29, 105, 122, 148, 157

Risk reduction, 47, 50, 58, 61, 65, 67, 68, 70, 71, 78, 92, 93, 95, 97, 98, 101, 104, 105, 106, 108, 109, 110, 111, 112, 113, 120, 123, 126, 139, 143, 146, 147, 149, 150, 153, 155, 156, 157, 158, 159, 161, 162
  condition, 58, 97, 98, 101, 106, 108, 111, 112, 120, 143, 153, 154
  formula, 61, 68, 92, 93, 101, 155
  model, 47, 50, 65, 67, 70, 71, 78, 95, 96, 97, 106, 108, 111, 112, 113, 120, 143, 150, 153, 156, 157, 159
Robins, 4, 8, 9

Schuckit, 16, 17, 53, 55, 56, 63, 87, 92, 93, 104, 105
Self-esteem, 42, 59, 68, 69, 72, 73, 77, 84, 99, 100, 125, 157
Social Development Model, 42, 80, 81, 83, 91, 92, 93, 111, 112, 113
Social factor, 10, 45, 51, 60, 65, 67, 69, 70, 91, 161, 162
Social Influences Model, 42, 73, 75, 77, 81, 112, 153
Social problem, 10, 46, 47, 49, 58, 60, 68, 69, 70, 101, 104, 114
Specificity, 102
Stanford University Three Communities Study, 31
STAR, 73, 74, 76, 112
Substance abuse, 1, 4, 24, 27, 45, 76, 101
Substances, 2, 3, 26, 29, 30, 35, 37, 45, 46, 49, 75, 77, 85, 90, 91, 109, 123, 143, 144, 151, 152, 153, 158, 159, 161
  differences between, 45, 153

Thompson, 62, 67, 90, 111, 126, 146
Tolerance, 27, 55, 56, 59, 68, 69, 92, 93, 104, 105, 126, 156
Tranquilizer, 3
Treatment, 25, 32, 63, 134
Trigger level, 51, 52, 68, 162
Twin, 54, 55, 129

Unambiguous expectation, 41
Unfreezing stage, 119, 120
Universal risk factor, 92

Use, 2, 3, 4, 5, 6, 7, 8, 9, 10, 11, 12, 13, 14,
        16, 17, 18, 19, 20, 21, 24, 25, 26, 27,
        28, 29, 30, 31, 32, 33, 34, 35, 36, 37,
        38, 39, 40, 41, 42, 43, 44, 45, 46, 47,
        49, 50, 57, 67, 68, 69, 70, 72, 73, 74,
        75, 76, 77, 78, 79, 80, 81, 82, 83, 84,
        85, 86, 88, 89, 90, 91, 92, 93, 94, 96,
        98, 99, 101, 102, 103, 105, 108, 110,
        111, 112, 114, 116, 118, 119, 123, 124,
        125, 126, 130, 131, 132, 134, 135,
        137, 138, 139, 140, 145, 147, 150,
        151, 152, 153, 154, 155, 156, 157,
        159, 160, 161, 162
    cause, 2, 4, 6, 21, 42, 43, 44, 46, 47, 50, 73,
        86, 88, 89, 151
    continuum, 44
    early, 4, 5, 6, 7, 8, 9, 10, 21, 79, 88, 89, 90,
        91, 153

Use (cont.)
    first, 2, 3, 4, 5, 6, 7, 8, 9, 10, 11, 73, 79, 86,
        88, 134
    high-risk, 16, 19, 20, 21, 26, 27, 32, 33, 34,
        35, 43, 44, 46, 69, 92, 105, 108, 116,
        119, 126, 145, 150, 151, 159, 161
    peer, 3, 7, 10, 11, 19, 21, 73, 74, 77, 80, 83,
        84, 90, 118, 135, 139
    responsible, 7, 14, 25, 26, 42, 160, 161
Use-related problem, 2, 4, 27, 28, 44, 46, 47,
        70, 93, 96, 101, 151

Vaillant, 62

War on Drugs, 18, 19
Wechsler, 13, 14, 16, 17
WHOA, 76
Wine cooler, 37, 38

About the Authors

Ray Daugherty has served as president of Prevention Research Institute Inc. (PRI) since 1984. Together with Terry O'Bryan, he cofounded PRI and coauthored eight curricula for prevention of, and intervention with, alcohol and drug problems, based on the Lifestyle Risk Reduction Model developed at PRI. Together, they guided the statewide implementation of DUI intervention programs in five states and national implementation of prevention programs for three collegiate fraternal organizations. Their curricula are in use at several hundred colleges throughout the United States and on selected U.S. Army installations in Europe and the United States. They also have worked for over 14 years with schools, parent organizations, and communities to prevent and interrupt alcohol and drug problems. Prior to his work with PRI, Ray served as executive director of the Kentucky Alcoholism Council, was founding director of a social setting detoxification center in Lexington, Kentucky, and helped establish the U.S. Army's alcohol and drug program at Camp Zama, Japan. He has lectured widely on theories and evaluation of prevention approaches.

Carl Leukefeld is a professor of psychiatry and behavioral science and director of the Drug and Alcohol Research Center at the University of Kentucky. He received his doctorate of social work from the Catholic University of America in 1975 and his master's degree at the University of Michigan. Before going to the University of

Kentucky, he was a commissioned officer in the U.S. Public Health Service and, for much of that time, was assigned to the National Institute on Drug Abuse in various clinical, management, and scientific capacities. He has coedited and written 15 books and monographs and has published over 80 articles and chapters.